Praise for *Beating Lyme: Understanding and Treating*
This Complex and Often Misdiagnosed Disease

"This searingly honest story of how medical politics today can block patient treatment and corrupt medical science must be read to be believed. It is also a glorious saga of how Lyme survivors and their doctors are challenging the status quo to help others recover. Bravo!"

—Norma Swenson, co-author, *Our Bodies, Ourselves*,
and faculty, Harvard School of Public Health

"This book should be read by anyone who has Lyme, suspects Lyme, or has an unexplained illness that physicians are ignoring. It is a condensed version of nearly everything that has happened regarding Lyme and tick-borne illnesses since 1993 and also includes the history of germs and vaccines from hundreds of years ago. We have never seen so much comprehensive information on the clinical and political aspects of Lyme disease and related disorders."

Linda Lobes, President,
The Michigan Lyme Disease Association

"An indispensable read for every medical student, physician, microbiologist, and victim of Lyme disease. One blueprint does not fit all, yet physicians are forced to follow a rigid protocol for a disease that acts like a defiant teen. Patients are considered collateral damage to those who set policy, while protecting profits, and physicians have to toe the line or else."

— Jim Wilson, President, The Canadian Lyme Disease Foundation

"You are either involved in treating it, know someone with it, or have it—"it" is Lyme disease. It is the most controversial disease, second most popular disease searched on the Internet, and it is the disease most likely to be misdiagnosed, undertreated, and underfunded. This is exactly why Constance Bean's book is so necessary to the Lyme disease community—worldwide. She has taken a twisted and complicated subject and made it understandable for everyone."

—Sue Vogan, host of *In Short Order*, an Internet radio show,
and author of *No Compassion Observed*

"I strongly endorse this book, which speaks forcefully for many of my patients who are unable to express themselves [about Lyme. Bean's] story speaks loud and clear for those who are suffering because the medical world remains divided, and many [patients] have even committed suicide rather than suffer a living hell. This is a must read for the public, Lyme patients, and the medical profession."

—Ernie Murakami, MD, Clinical Associate Professor Emeritus,
University of British Columbia Medical School Department
of Family Practice, special interest, Lyme disease

P9-CSW-583

"This book would be helpful for any patient who wants a comprehensive overview of Lyme, from the historical viewpoint to an in-depth look at the problems that continue to plague diagnosis and treatment."

—Phyllis Mervine, Founder and President,
California Lyme Disease Association

"*Beating Lyme* is an excellent narrative on the history of a painful, debilitating infection called Lyme disease. The author provides important information about the disease itself and the complex political issues that are causing tremendous and needless suffering in patients throughout the United States. This is a much-anticipated book that will educate the reader and increase public awareness of a dangerous and growing infectious disease epidemic. As a Lyme patient and Founder/President of the Lyme Education Awareness Program, L.E.A.P. Arizona, I am thankful to Constance Bean for sharing her personal experience with Lyme disease and for her willingness to pull back the curtain for a behind-the-scenes look at this American medical and insurance tragedy."

—Tina Garcia, Founder/President,
Lyme Education Awareness Program (L.E.A.P.), Arizona

"This publication is one more brick in the wall of truth about this debilitating and insidious disease that is wreaking havoc on our nation and the world, while the powers-that-be pretend it is less of a danger than the common cold. It is a highly recommended read that should be mandatory for all doctors."

—Randy Sykes, co-founder,
The Greater Hartford Lyme Disease Foundation

"One may ask, 'What could possibly be worse than suffering with a disease that still remains a hushed and hidden epidemic?' The answer is, 'The plague of ignorance that surrounds it.' An absolute must read with benefits for us all, now and for generations to come."

—Tracie Schlissel and Leslie Wermers,
(two sisters diagnosed with late-stage Lyme),
co-founders, The Minnesota Lyme Fighters Advocacy

Also by Constance A. Bean

Methods of Childbirth

Labor and Delivery, An Observer's Diary

Methods of Childbirth, rev. ed.

The Better Back Book

Methods of Childbirth: The Completely Updated Version of a Classic Work for Today's Woman, rev. ed.

Women Murdered by the Men They Loved (Haworth Women's Studies)

BEATING LYME

Understanding and Treating This Complex and Often Misdiagnosed Disease

Constance A. Bean

with Lesley Ann Fein, M.D., M.P.H.

AMACOM

American Management Association
New York • Atlanta • Brussels • Chicago • Mexico City • San Francisco
Shanghai • Tokyo • Toronto • Washington, D.C.

Special discounts on bulk quantities of AMACOM books are
available to corporations, professional associations, and other
organizations. For details, contact Special Sales Department,
AMACOM, a division of American Management Association,
1601 Broadway, New York, NY 10019.
Tel.: 212-903-8316.   Fax: 212-903-8083.
E-mail: specialsls@amanet.org
Website: www.amacombooks.org/go/specialsales
To view all AMACOM titles go to: www.amacombooks.org

*This publication is designed to provide accurate and authoritative information in regard to the subject
matter covered. It is sold with the understanding that the publisher is not engaged in rendering legal,
accounting, or other professional service. If legal advice or other expert assistance is required, the services
of a competent professional person should be sought.*

Grateful acknowledgment is made to the following, who granted permission to reprint material in this book:
The American Lyme Disease Foundation, for the pictures. **Contingencies** Irwin Vanderhoof, PhD, CLU
et al, "Lyme Disease: The Cost to Society," Jan/Feb 1993. **New York Times** Lawrence Altman, "Annual
Exam Gives Bush Good Marks for Health," August 9, 1997; David Grann, "Stalking Dr. Steere," New
York Times Magazine, June 17, 2001; Holcomb Noble, "Questioning Long-Term Lyme Disease," May 23,
2000, "Lyme Doctors Rally Behind a Colleague Under Inquiry," November 10, 2000, "Concerns Grow
Over Reaction to Lyme Shot," November 21, 2000; "Lyme Disease Is Hard to Catch, Easy to Halt," June
13, 2001. **Newsweek** David France, "War Against Doctors," November 11, 2000; Mary Carmichael, "The
Great Lyme Debate," August 6, 2007. **Pediatrics** Henry M. Feder and Jr., MD, "Differences Are Voiced
by Two Lyme Camps at a Connecticut Public Hearing on Insurance Coverage of Lyme Disease," no. 105,
pp. 855-857. **Yankee Magazine** Edie Clark, "Trouble in Paradise," July/August 2007.

Library of Congress Cataloging-in-Publication Data

Bean, Constance A.
  Beating Lyme : understanding and treating this complex and often misdiagnosed disease /
Constance A. Bean with Lesley Ann Fein.
      p.   cm.
   Includes bibliographical references and index.
   ISBN-13: 978-0-8144-0944-2
   ISBN-10: 0-8144-0944-X
   1. Lyme disease—Popular works.   I. Fein, Lesley Ann.   II. Title.

RC155.5.B43 2008
616.9′246—dc22
          2008012699

Printing number

10   9   8   7   6   5   4   3   2   1

This book is dedicated to all who have struggled to find medical treatment for Lyme disease and to the Lyme organizations and support groups that work to prevent this from happening to others. It is dedicated to doctors who do not dismiss those who are sometimes desperately ill but provide the individualized treatment that may be necessary to return their Lyme patients to normal lives.

Contents

Contents

PREFACE

Beating Lyme covers the fascinating, yet completely trivialized, relationship between infections, and the consequences of the chronic pain syndrome that inevitably ensues when Lyme disease is not correctly diagnosed.

My interest in this field of medicine stems from my fascination with the ability of the bacterial and viral organisms to inhabit the human body, yet not destroy it. These infections set up an environment for themselves that enhances their survival, yet does not kill the host.

Borrelia burgdorferi (Bb) enters the body via the skin, travels to local nerves and lymphatic channels, penetrates the blood stream, and can rapidly invade the brain without the host even knowing. Bb has been isolated from the spinal fluid of victims hours after a tick bite when the host is completely asymptomatic!

It then sets up house inside cells, evades detection, but also starts playing games with the immune system. In some people it causes nonspecific activation of all immune cells resulting in a clinical presentation that looks exactly like lupus or rheumatoid arthritis (RA), and many other autoimmune diseases, including sarcoidosis, multiple sclerosis, Parkinson's, ALS, and lupus.

In these people, whom I affectionately call "Balb C mice (those who develop lupus when infected with Lyme and have negative testing for Lyme serologies), we need to treat both the infection and the manifestations. Sometimes the autoimmune diseases are so extreme that all weapons, including steroids, embrel, i.v. gammaglobulin, Plaquenil, and so on, must be used to stop it while also trying to rid Lyme sufferers of the underlying infection at the same time. This is a very delicate balance, yet one that fascinates me the most.

How do we suppress the "anti-self" antibodies and also keep the immune system intact enough to get rid of all the bugs at the same time? Can we undo the damage that has already been done in diseases such as MS and ALS? Is it sometimes too late? The answer, sadly, is yes. Anti-self antibodies attack your own tissues instead of foreign invaders. These antibodies create inflammation and pain in joints and tissues because they are confusing your own cells as foreign.

We must understand and address the role that the Th 1 pathway (which initiates immune responses) plays in patients who have very high 1,25D/25 Vitamin D ratios. The inactive form is 25 D; the active form is 1,25 D. Vitamin D is considered vital in immune pathways.) In the Th1 inflammatory diseases, excessive amounts of Vitamin D cause inflammation and allow activation of multiple other bacteria and viruses that are in dormant states. Our bodies are always living in harmony with bacteria and viruses until something comes along to ruin the homeostasis.

I hypothesize that chronic Lyme creates the perfect environment in some people for activation of bacteria and viruses associated with chronic fatigue syndrome.

We now have people whom I affectionately call "cess pools," and it is our job to figure out which bug is winning the game and start attacking that one first, or immediately attack both the bacteria and viruses which are identified. It is known that EBV (Epstein Barr Virus causing mononucleosis) and Bb (Borrelia burgdorferi causing Lyme) promote each other's survival. We will not conquer one without attacking the other. We know bacteria such as Mycoplasma, Bartonella, and Chlamydia pneumonia play a huge role in these chronic infections. We must, therefore, attack each one at some point in the treatment program. We also need to decide if CMV (cytomegalovirus), Parvovirus, and HHV6 (a subgroup of herpes viruses) are affecting the host. If they are, we need to address them. I have learned a lot from the extensive research in CFS (Chronic Fatigue Syndrome, now called CFSME with ME standing for myeloencephelopathy), and we must use all the knowledge they have unearthed to help us treat those with Lyme, including the many studies on the value of specific supplements.

I need to address the often unjustified fear of long-term antibiotics. Why do we not care that our kids are on tetracyclines for years for acne? The side effects are minimal as long as the doctor is monitoring diet, acidophilus, and blood tests. Patients who trade off getting better with long-term antibiotics and staying disabled do not think twice. We deal with side effects and move on. Since it is well documented that untreated Lyme suppresses the immune system, I argue that when we treat for as long as it takes to achieve remission, we strengthen the immune system.

Do we know that there are resistant strains? Yes. Do we know that Lyme can develop resistance in humans? No. We do know that it changes its shape from a motile bacterium into a cell wall deficient form, which sits inside cells and can secrete a protective coat to "cloak" itself. We also know there are hundreds of different strains. Do we test for all of them? No. Do some tests miss most of them? Definitely.

Finally, studies have shown that virtually everyone with chronic pain syndrome ends up having Fibromyalgia. After your brain has been bombarded with substance P for long enough, your inhibitory neurons finally give up and run out of serotonin. (Substance P is made by the pain center in the spinal cord when the center receives pain signals. It tells the brain there is pain. In chronic pain syndromes, the inhibitory interneurons get depleted of serotonin and stop doing their job of blunting pain signals.) You now officially have Fibromyalgia. Every sensory input is not blunted. You react to light, touch, sounds, have sleep disruption, get irritable and moody, and cannot concentrate because your brain is in overload. You have to leave stores with high lighting because you can't stand the lights and the noise. Your brain is screaming to be protected from all this input because the serotonin fibers have stopped protecting your brain by filtering background noise. These issues must be addressed and fixed if you are ever to return to normal.

Sleep is mandatory to allow your immune system to recharge and make growth hormone. Do not be afraid to take medications to help you sleep! I tell my patients that martyrdom does not promote healing. Treat the pain. Treat the sleep disorder. Take tryptophane and SSRI's. Protect your brain from unnecessary input. Accept the fact that your brain is "in charge" of your body and you must let it perform its "normal" functions if you are to get better.

It saddens me that so few physicians refuse to deal with these complicated Lyme patients. Granted, they take a lot of work and dedication to fix, but when they are better, there is no finer sense of gratification. Is this due to the fact that insurance companies refuse to pay for our time? Probably. There is no way you can deal with all of these problems in a $60 visit. Is it insurance companies refusing to pay for tests and treatment? Definitely. In my office, Regina spends every day trying to authorize medications down to simple ones that we never had to justify before! Is it large groups like the IDSA and Neurology association actively trivializing this complex illness? Definitely. The question is why? What is their motivation? Are they truly clueless? Do they not care to get involved? Of course, it is the safe approach. Are they concerned about repercussions? Of course! How many of us have been exposed to harassment and hearings? Most of us! Are we dumb to keep holding the torch? Maybe. Do they have a large financial stake in denying the existence of these diseases? Definitely. Look at the money received by "experts" for insurance companies, and the money from patenting vaccines and then testing kits that evolve from the vaccines, which then earn millions.

I can only speak for myself. I love what I do. I love figuring out the puzzle and slowly solving it. I am grateful to work with a group of brilliant physicians and therapists, and deeply mourn the loss of Drs.

Preface

Hamlin and Bleiweiss. John Bleiweiss was an internist and aggressive treater of Lyme. He was charged by the New Jersey Board of Medical Examiners with inappropriate diagnosis and treatment for this disease. He ended his life after being unable to endure the stress. Carey Hamilton was a psychiatrist who found abnormal areas of electrical activity in most of the temporal lobes in the brains of his Lyme patients. He died unexpectedly before publishing his work.

I love transforming people from wheelchairs, crying all the time, to active healthy people. Nothing warms the heart more when you are a doctor to hear the words, "Doc, you saved my life!" No. I will not stop. I will always try to learn as much as I can. I will fight with insurance companies. I will argue with the doctors who tell me there is "no such thing as..." My oath and my conscience leave me with no choice.

I bless this author for uncovering these issues, and I beg the medical profession to start looking at these diseases more closely. When you do, you will feel as I do, and enjoy the slow trudge up that high mountain of recovery!

—Lesley Ann Fein, MD, MPH

---

*It has recently been uncovered that if the ratio between 1, 25D (active D) and 25D (inactive D) is greater than 1.5 that person has an inflammatory reaction to underlying infections seen in sarcoidosis and crohn's disease, and probably Lyme and CFS. The ratio between 1, 25D and 25 D is supposed to be 1.5 or less. If it is higher than 1.5, it implies Th 1 inflammation which has been associated with chronic intracellular infections.

ACKNOWLEDGMENTS

S cience and clinical experience tell us that Lyme is an infectious disease that if untreated can progress. Yet we continue to have the disease unrecognized to the point where it is misdiagnosed with every condition from chronic fatigue to Alzheimer's. Patients who have symptoms are told they don't have Lyme. Doctors have visited their Lyme patients in the hospital to find that the antibiotics they have ordered have been withdrawn by another doctor because "the patient doesn't need them any longer."

Dr. Sam T. Donta, well-known infectious disease physician with years of experience and published papers on Lyme disease, diagnosed and treated my disease. Without his careful attention my situation would have remained dire.

Dr. Lesley Ann Fein came on board. She has long understood the Lyme disease treatment problem, and I am pleased that she is part of this book. Her daughter, Amanda Kay Norwich, reviewed the book, and I thank her.

Robert Spallone of New Jersey, then a counselor in Lyme disease, offered information and support that were essential when I was seriously ill. From him I learned the politics of Lyme and the importance of "hanging in."

Sue Vogan, journalist, author, and radio show host, shared her extensive knowledge and provided invaluable information and support for this book. She is a resource beyond measure.

Acknowledgments

Many individuals, groups, and associations offer ongoing education and support for those who are ill. I acknowledge the work of those who maintain the Lyme disease websites on serious illness.

Robert Shuman, my editor at AMACOM, saw the importance of this book within days of receiving it. Bob, also editor of two of my previous books, was a delight to work with, providing ongoing support and close attention to every detail throughout the process. He offered wise counsel for this book on a story that is largely unknown.

CHAPTER ONE

THE HIDDEN EPIDEMIC

*Someone in my office had Lyme disease and has recovered. I've heard that
you can get quite sick with it. How do you know whether you have it and
what should you do? I've seen quite a few ticks in my yard.*

—AUDIENCE MEMBER AT A LOCAL
GARDEN CLUB MEETING ON LYME DISEASE

Many people who get Lyme disease are given an antibiotic and
then have no further concern about the disease; within a few
weeks they can expect to be cured. Here's what happened to Tom: He
awoke one day feeling unusually tired. During the following days he felt
mildly ill and occasionally somewhat lightheaded. He noticed a red area
on his arm that he could not explain. Still not feeling well, he called his
doctor, who asked if he could have been bitten by a tick. After learning
that Tom had played golf the preceding weekend and searched for balls
in long grass and brush, his doctor suspected Tom could have been exposed to Lyme disease and took no chances. He prescribed four weeks
of an antibiotic and said, "Call if you're still not feeling well." At the end
of the month, Tom had no more bouts of fatigue or further worries
about the disease. There are no guarantees, but the information contained in this book helps assure that this will be the case for you.

Even with delayed medical help, most people will still recover from
Lyme, but Lisa did not fare quite as well as Tom. She was bitten by a

deer tick in a heavily infested area north of Boston. Her Lyme test, however, was negative, and she was not given an antibiotic. "Within a few weeks I had shooting pains in my legs and one of them swelled up. My primary care doctor sent me to an orthopedist, who says I have arthritis that will get worse. I may end up in a wheelchair. I'm only 35 years old, a single mother with two young children. How can I have suddenly come down with arthritis? How can this be?" She was in tears and already nearly unable to walk.

She contacted a second orthopedist, who supported the earlier opinion given that she had arthritis. She asked for another Lyme test, which also came back negative. The second doctor said the Lyme tests done at the hospital were very accurate, so she prepared for a life of invalidism. She resigned from her computer job and abandoned plans for an advanced degree. Since her mother lived in faraway Japan, Lisa contacted social agencies for help in caring for herself and her children and looked into her eligibility for disability payments. The future seemed to hold little except invalidism and pain. After several weeks of despair, she sought further information. By making more phone calls, she learned of a doctor with experience in treating Lyme disease. She waited for the appointment date to arrive and only then discovered that she did indeed have the infection. After three months of antibiotic treatment, she became well and remains healthy, but her story could have been very different.

Medical care for Lyme disease remains remarkably unavailable for those who are not treated promptly after the bite of an infected deer tick. This book tells you why and provides information that will help you avoid the risks that many take without knowing what they are. With facts in hand, it becomes possible to find help, whether to preserve or to recover your health after being bitten by a tick. We don't yet have all the answers, but there are choices that allow you to decide on the degree of risk that you are willing to accept.

The story of Lyme disease and how it is diagnosed and treated is presented in this book. Here I'll also delineate the controversy and politics that play the major role in denying its presence and obstructing treatment. My disease, for example, was not recognized, and I had the experience of thousands of others as I struggled to find medical care. I learned the nearly unbelievable politics that stood in the way of finding help. Although this is not a personal saga, at intervals I'll describe what happened to me, how I coped, and the medical treatment that I was fortunate to receive.

EXPLODING NUMBERS OF TICKS AND LYME DISEASE

Lyme disease has become increasingly prevalent during the past few years, occurring very far from East Coast states where it was originally discovered. (See Figure 1-1.) It is the fastest-growing infectious disease in America, and some of its victims become either mildly or severely ill. In 1993, 8,257 new cases were reported. In the year 2000, 17,730 cases were reported. In 2005, there were 23,305 new cases reported, approximately three times as many as in 1991. The numbers climb, conservatively, at least 8 percent per year. In Europe approximately 60,000 cases are reported annually, and the numbers are increasing in Canada. There is Lyme disease in Great Britain, Sweden, Finland, and Asia. It has become a global disease.

No one knows how much Lyme disease there actually is because many cases are never recognized or aren't diagnosed until months or years later. And many cases that are diagnosed are never reported to a state's department of public health. Reporting depends on physician initiative, and physicians often don't send information, especially if they're unsure whether their patient has Lyme disease. It is inevitable that many cases are missed.

When national reporting began in 1982, there were 497 cases reported. In 1992 it was mandated. The data collection policy is determined by state laws or regulations, which may differ in each state. Information is received from licensed health care providers, local health departments, diagnostic laboratories, or hospitals. This data from states and the District of Columbia is shared with the Centers for

State	1993	1994	1995	1996	1997	1998	1999	2000	2001	2002	2003	2004	2005	2006	Incidence 2006*
Alabama	4	6	12	9	11	24	20	6	10	11	8	6	3	11	0.2
Alaska	0	0	0	0	2	1	0	2	2	3	3	3	4	3	0.4
Arizona	0	0	1	0	4	1	3	2	3	4	4	13	10	10	0.2
Arkansas	8	15	11	27	27	8	7	7	4	3	0	0	0	0	0.0
California	134	68	84	64	154	135	139	96	95	97	86	48	95	85	0.2
Colorado	0	1	0	0	0	0	3	0	0	1	0	0	0	0	0.0
Connecticut	1350	2030	1548	3104	2297	3434	3215	3773	3597	4631	1403	1348	1810	1788	51.0
Delaware	143	106	56	173	109	77	167	167	152	194	212	339	646	482	56.5
DC	2	9	3	3	10	8	6	11	17	25	14	16	10	62	10.7
Florida	30	28	17	55	56	71	59	54	43	79	43	46	47	34	0.2
Georgia	44	127	14	1	9	5	0	0	0	2	10	12	6	8	0.1
Hawaii	1	0	0	1	0	0	0	0	0	0	0	0	0	0	0.0
Idaho	2	3	0	2	4	7	3	4	5	4	3	6	2	7	0.5
Illinois	19	24	18	10	13	14	17	35	32	47	71	87	127	110	0.9
Indiana	32	19	19	32	33	39	21	23	26	21	25	32	33	26	0.4
Iowa	8	17	16	19	8	27	24	34	36	42	58	49	89	97	3.3
Kansas	54	17	23	36	4	13	16	17	2	7	4	3	3	4	0.1
Kentucky	16	24	16	26	20	27	19	13	23	25	17	15	5	7	0.2
Louisiana	3	4	9	9	13	15	9	8	8	5	7	2	3	1	0.0
Maine	18	33	45	63	34	78	41	71	108	219	175	225	247	338	25.6
Maryland	180	341	454	447	494	659	899	688	608	738	691	891	1235	1248	22.2
Massachusetts	148	247	189	321	291	699	787	1158	1164	1807	1532	1532	2336	1432	22.2
Michigan	23	33	5	28	27	17	11	23	21	26	12	27	62	55	0.5
Minnesota	141	208	208	251	256	261	283	465	461	867	474	1023	917	914	17.7

4

State															cases per 100,000 population
Mississippi	0	0	17	24	27	17	4	3	8	12	21	0	0	3	0.1
Missouri	108	102	53	52	28	12	72	47	37	41	70	25	15	5	0.1
Montana	0	0	0	0	0	0	0	0	4	0	0	0	0	1	0.1
Nebraska	6	3	6	5	2	4	11	8	4	6	2	2	2	11	0.6
Nevada	5	1	6	2	2	6	2	4	4	2	3	1	3	4	0.2
New Hampshire	15	30	28	47	39	45	27	84	129	261	190	226	265	617	46.9
New Jersey	786	1533	1703	2190	2041	1911	1719	2459	2020	2349	2887	2698	3363	2432	27.9
New Mexico	2	5	1	1	1	4	1	0	1	1	1	1	3	3	0.2
New York	2818	5200	4438	5301	3327	4640	4402	4329	4083	5535	5399	5100	5565	4460	23.1
Oklahoma	19	99	63	42	45	13	8	1	0	0	0	3	0	0	0.0
Oregon	8	6	20	19	20	21	15	13	15	12	16	11	3	7	0.2
Pennsylvania	1085	1438	1562	2814	2188	2760	2781	2343	2606	3989	5730	3985	4287	3242	26.1
Rhode Island	272	471	345	534	442	789	546	675	510	852	736	249	39	308	28.8
South Carolina	9	7	17	9	3	8	6	25	6	26	18	22	15	20	0.5
South Dakota	0	0	0	0	1	0	0	0	0	2	1	1	2	1	0.1
Tennessee	20	13	28	24	45	47	59	28	31	28	20	20	8	15	0.2
Texas	48	56	77	97	60	32	72	77	75	139	85	98	69	29	0.1
Utah	2	3	1	1	1	0	2	3	-	5	2	1	2	5	0.2
Vermont	12	16	9	26	8	11	26	40	18	37	43	50	54	105	16.8
Virginia	95	131	55	57	67	73	122	149	156	259	195	216	274	357	4.7
Washington	9	4	10	18	11	7	14	9	9	11	7	14	13	8	0.1
West Virginia	50	29	26	12	10	13	20	35	16	26	31	38	61	28	1.5
Wisconsin	401	409	369	396	480	657	490	631	597	1090	740	1144	1459	1466	26.4
Wyoming	9	5	4	3	3	1	3	3	1	2	2	4	3	1	0.2
U.S. TOTAL	8,257	13,043	11,700	16,455	12,801	16,801	16,273	17,730	17,029	23,763	21,273	19,804	23,305	19,931	8.24

* cases per 100,000 population

Figure 1-1. Reported Cases by State, 1993–2006.

5

Disease Control (CDC). Because of recent budget cuts, Connecticut laboratories, for example, are no longer required to report Lyme disease.

The actual figure is estimated by all sources, including the government, to be at least ten times the recorded numbers. With this number in mind, 230,000 Americans may have contracted Lyme disease, and some experts estimate that as many as 1.7 million may be infected with Lyme bacteria. At a legislative hearing in Albany, New York, on November 27, 2001, it was estimated that at least 10,000 people in New York were living with chronic Lyme disease.

Lyme disease is no longer confined to Cape Cod, Connecticut, the northeastern and mid-Atlantic states, and the Great Lakes region. For a variety of reasons, which include more people moving into forested areas, climate warming, and increasing numbers of deer and deer ticks, it has spread across the United States and is found in nearly every continental state. It is a recognized problem in Virginia, the Carolinas, Georgia, and Missouri. It is prevalent in the state of Washington and in several parts of California, and has become an increasing problem in Maine, Vermont, and New Hampshire. You cannot be assured of safety from Lyme even in urban areas, including New York City parks. States reporting the most cases are Connecticut, New York, Pennsylvania, Rhode Island, and Wisconsin. Most of these are reported in the late summer, but the disease is reported in every month of the year. (See Figure 1-2.) If you are visiting or traveling in any state and take a walk in fields, brush, or woods, you are at risk of encountering a disease-carrying tick.

The risk to the public increases as more deer ticks become infected, making every tick bite of greater concern. In 2000 researchers at the Portland, Maine, Lyme Disease Research Laboratory found that the infection rate of ticks was about 30 percent. Four years later, out of every hundred ticks collected at Crescent Beach Park, fifty-five were infected with Lyme disease. Infection rates at Cape Elizabeth, Kittery, and Wells are now greater than 50 percent. As many as a third, and, in many cases, far more of the ticks in New York, Massachusetts, Connecticut, Delaware, Rhode Island, and New Jersey are infected with

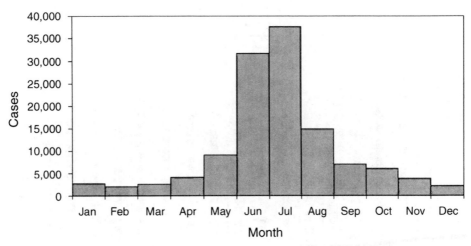

Figure 1-2. Reported Cases of Lyme Disease by Month of Illness Onset
United States, 1992–2004.

Lyme. The risk of West Nile virus or pandemic flu can't compare with
the current risk of Lyme. If this illness were associated in any way with
bioterrorism, the response would be very different.

The age groups most affected are children from 5 to 14 and adults
over a wide range, beginning at age 30. More specifically, the CDC
says that although people of all ages are susceptible to tick bite, Lyme
disease is most common among boys 5 to 19 years old and people 30
and up. (See Figure 1-3.)

How Serious Is Lyme?

The disease can be incredibly easy to acquire, and the ticks that transmit it are just as likely to be found in suburban yards as they are in
woods and fields, or among coastal bushes and beach grass. With the
possible exception of being transmitted through pregnancy, Lyme is
acquired only from a bite from an infected tick. Many cases of the
disease are so mild, as one woman says, "It could be Lyme disease but
I can live with it." In most cases it is cured within a few weeks, even
when symptoms have developed beyond the early rash and bacteria
have spread to the brain, causing fatigue, dizziness, and malaise.

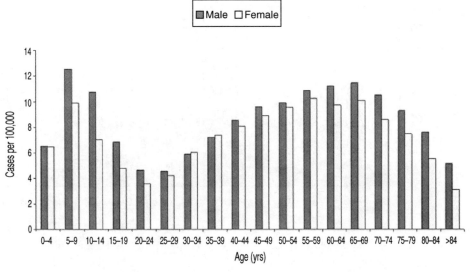

Figure 1-3. Average Annual Incidence of Reported Cases of Lyme Disease by Age Group and Sex, United States, 1992–2004.

Even people who remain undiagnosed for months, or years, can recover. When they are given adequate treatment, many return to work and normal lives. Every case is different, and we don't yet have all the answers, but we do know that even late-stage disabling Lyme disease responds to antibiotic treatment. The information provided here will help you avoid serious illness, which has affected thousands who were bitten by an infected tick.

My story is typical of many whose Lyme disease is not recognized early and treated adequately. What happened to me continues to happen to others. I became ill in May 1993 and was not diagnosed until December of that year, a time period far shorter than that for most who acquire serious disease. If I had known then what I learned later, I might have found treatment sooner. I read books that told me about ticks but gave no answers to my dilemma. I was trying to get diagnosed; I knew it had to be Lyme disease, every other illness was ruled out. I didn't know why I wasn't treated or what the treatment should be. I had no idea one could get so sick with Lyme and why the doctors didn't know what I had. As yet, I didn't know about the contro-versy that gets in the way of doctors' diagnosing the disease. Though Lyme disease was identified in 1975, information on untreated Lyme remains largely unavailable, and the number of those with unrecog-nized disease continues to remain generally unknown to the public and to physicians.

MY EXPERIENCE IN GETTING DIAGNOSED

I lay in bed with a flulike illness, a pink rash spreading across the back of my hip. I didn't know it then, but the bite of a tiny insect, no big-ger than a poppy seed, had changed my life. Several weeks earlier, while at my Cape Cod vacation home, I discovered a small deer tick burrowed into the back of my hip and firmly attached. With the help of a small magnifying glass I saw that it appeared to have legs and rushed to the nearby medical center to have it removed. Soon after the tick was removed, the skin around the bite became red, and I re-turned to the medical center the following day.

The physician suggested that the rash could be caused by an allergy to the Band-Aid, perhaps part of the tick remained under the skin, or it might be due to an infection. He said, "You must be allergic to some-thing in the Band-Aid. It isn't Lyme disease." Though allergies to la-tex bandages are not uncommon, this didn't apply to me. I assured him I was allergic to absolutely nothing, certainly not to a bandage. He gave me, just as a precaution, in case I did have an infection of some kind, a two-week antibiotic prescription which I filled at the nearest phar-macy. I returned to my home near Boston, unsuspecting of the com-ing nightmare. I became part of the hidden epidemic, ignored by medical science, that leaves victims untreated. Even the fact that they are sick is often unrecognized. I had never before been ill and had no medical records anywhere. Soon it seemed that I had medical records almost everywhere.

At the end of two weeks, my face was flushed, and sometimes my souvenir Jamaican t-shirts were soaked with sweat. The rash continued to spread in all directions. I raced the hundred miles back to the medical center for a prescription refill, where I discovered that the protocol from Boston's New England Medical Center was two weeks of antibiotic treatment. Staff members said they could give no more.

I looked at the doctor and nurse, my eyes wide and questioning. Obviously, whatever my problem was, it hadn't resolved. My background is in public health, and I didn't know why my antibiotic was limited to two weeks. The staff was doing what it had been told. "We're following the protocol," explained the nurse. When it became clear that I wasn't leaving without explanation or prescription, I was given a two-week refill. If I had been even remotely exposed to anthrax, in a heartbeat I would have been given this same drug long term, not just for two weeks. Medical science has yet to recognize that Lyme disease is a complex disease that may require longer treatment and the use of a variety of antibiotics.

It would be a while before I discovered that the disease is controversial, and that other tick-borne diseases are also carried by the same tick that carries Lyme bacteria. Because I then, like most people even now, was ignorant of the controversy, I didn't know my risk of chronic disease, but common sense raised my concerns. Even though from the time the disease was identified, it was known that the bite of an infected deer tick could have serious arthritic and neurological consequences, the medical staff appeared puzzlingly unconcerned, despite the fact that Cape Cod has one of the highest rates of Lyme disease in the United States.

MY SEARCH FOR HELP

My world began to close around me. I was not getting better. My neck ached all the time and I had a constant mild headache. My shoulder hurt, and sometimes I had minor muscle pains. I felt lightheaded. At my visit with a recently trained internist, I told him about my tick bite, showed him my slowly fading rash, and asked about Lyme disease. I reported that I had been on an antibiotic briefly, in case I had the disease. He said my problem was not Lyme disease and to get off the antibiotic immediately. "If you had the disease, it has already been cured with the antibiotic and you should get off the medicine right away. It could be causing your symptoms. Too much antibiotic can be harmful." This statement appeared irrelevant to my situation, but I followed his advice.

The physician ordered a shoulder X-ray and handed me samples of muscle relaxants from his desk drawer, suggesting that I might have a virus. "Come back for a physical exam, perhaps in six months, when you are feeling better." He didn't know the meaning of my symptoms or my test results. My blood tests, including the Lyme disease test, checked out normal. I asked for a repeat of the Lyme test, and again the result came back negative, as it often does for this disease. The internist and I seemingly had nowhere to go for either diagnosis or treatment. We didn't know that the usual blood tests are typically normal for those with Lyme disease, or that the Lyme test that is usually given is as problematical as the treatment. We didn't know about the disease that had progressed beyond early flulike symptoms and was rapidly disabling me.

This was my second experience facing the consequences of the Lyme disease controversy. I went home and back to bed, continuing to be puzzled by the treatment limitation and lack of acknowledgment of my illness, the tick bite cause of which seemed obvious to me. Only a little more than two months earlier I had been well while traveling with my husband in England.

I continued my search for help. One Sunday morning nine weeks after the tick had been removed I made the first of several trips to a hospital emergency room. I had a mild fever and felt an occasional curious threadlike pain in one knee. I told my story to the emergency room physician at the Metrowest Medical Center in Framingham and asked for an antibiotic. He sat with pen in hand, poised to write the prescription. However, when I mentioned I had already been given four weeks of antibiotics he put down his pen, somewhat reluctantly

I thought, and said, "If this is Lyme disease, you've already had enough treatment." He suggested seeing an infectious disease expert. "We have a Lyme disease specialist on staff, but he's on a trip to Japan." I learned later that this doctor is among those who believe that Lyme disease is overdiagnosed and overtreated.

During ensuing months I saw at least three infectious disease specialists in the Boston area. All offered neither acknowledgment of my disease nor treatment for it. Mine is not a unique story, or one that happens only to a few. It is the norm for thousands whose disease is not recognized and treated early.

THE LYME DISEASE CLINIC

By the time I went for my appointment at the Lyme disease clinic at the New England Medical Center in Boston, one knee was swollen and I still had the rash, but the two physicians who dashed into the examining room were quick to announce that it wasn't Lyme. They stayed in the examining room for less than thirty seconds. I was dismissed without referral or follow-up. It is a common experience that when a condition is perceived as outside the disease-labeling norms, or is considered psychosomatic, sufferers are left with nothing.

The clinic was headed by Dr. Allen Steere, a rheumatologist who first identified Lyme disease in 1975 and a chief proponent of the theory that Lyme disease is overdiagnosed and overtreated. He was the lead author of the 2000 Infectious Diseases Society of America (IDSA) guidelines recommending limitations on Lyme disease diagnosis and treatment. I didn't know about the guidelines, and I could not have understood them even if I had known. The question continues, "How can they leave patients untreated and sick?"

At a rheumatology appointment at the same hospital, the physician noted weakness in my arms and legs. When I walked along the hall, I wasn't picking up my feet. When he pushed against my arms, I had trouble pushing back. "Your record says you don't have Lyme disease," he said with some apparent doubt. He suggested a computerized axial tomography (CAT) scan of my chest, in case I had a tumor, and asked that I attend an endocrinologists' case review meeting. I had the CAT scan, accepting radiation that I didn't want. The nurse who accompanied me to radiology said quietly, "I think you have Lyme."

Books fell out of my hands. At a second emergency room trip, this time to the New England Medical Center, I was nearly unable to walk from the parking lot. I crouched in a corner of the busy waiting room, my head between my knees. My blood pressure was way below normal. A few minutes later the nurse checked again and this time the reading was considerably higher than it should be. She said, "You can't trust these blood pressure readings." I was shivering. A CAT scan of my head was ordered in case I had a neurological problem, such as a possible brain tumor. Still no diagnosis. At 2:00 a.m. on that hot summer night, as I limped from the emergency room entrance to the hospital parking lot across the street, a half-dozen women wearing short skirts and gold chains strolled in front of the entrance. I envied them their mobility.

MORE HOSPITAL TRIPS

Only days later, a racing, pounding heart along with weakness and my other symptoms sent me to the Lahey Clinic emergency room in Burlington, Massachusetts. Having no transportation on such short notice, and not daring to drive the distance, I went by ambulance. I sat up during the trip. Once there, I walked into the emergency room, not needing the stretcher. The staff did not know why I was there. To them, I didn't look sick.

A couple of days later a second episode with a pounding heart and irregular heartbeat sent me back to the same emergency room where I was given a twenty-four-hour heart monitor. The staff did not know that a racing, pounding heart is one of the possible Lyme disease symptoms. Many Lyme patients have in their records the twenty-four-hour heart monitor. The test was negative, showing no heart abnormalities. When I asked about the possibility of Lyme disease, I was told that if I had ever had the disease I had already recovered.

The Lahey Clinic is a world-famous medical facility, and I sought its help. I spent a day at the hospital, seeing a series of specialists. I remember a spacious, carpeted lobby, furnished with many upholstered chairs, and with lots of light coming through large areas of glass. I recall the corridors as wide and also carpeted. I saw the world through a bright haze and blinked my eyes against the light. I struggled to walk the corridors to the physician offices.

I now had multiple rashes on my neck and chest which the dermatologist could not identify, but he was unconcerned. His manner was rushed and he seemed irritable. Why is this woman at the famed Lahey Clinic for a few red spots on her neck? He didn't know about Lyme disease rashes, or that the disease could be serious. Mine were not the oft-described bull's-eye rash with a red dot in the center. The rashes weren't even located where I had been bitten, on the back of my hip. Multiple rashes far from the bite site are common during the course of disseminated Lyme disease, but nothing in this physician's training prepared him to help me.

He passed me on to the hematologist. This doctor was concerned, thinking the rashes might be caused by a blood-clotting disorder. He scheduled tests and another visit. But he was trained to see the symptom through the lens of his own specialty and could not recognize the rashes as a symptom of Lyme disease. The test results were negative for a clotting disorder.

I thought the rheumatologist might understand my painful knees. He bent over my records while talking fast and nonstop, about what I cannot recall, but it wasn't about getting me diagnosed. He noted that my records said I didn't have Lyme disease. My recollection is that he asked few, if any, questions and that I was given no chance to talk, but I can't be sure because I felt so very sick. The focus didn't seem to be on me and why I was there. On his desk was a picture of a row of healthy, smiling women in colorful gowns, perhaps at a party or wedding. Their world seemed very far from what mine had become, the world of illness.

I climbed onto an examining table that appeared impossibly high. Lying on the hard table, every muscle and bone seemed to hurt. To my surprise, the rheumatologist didn't mention my swollen knees. My knee and chest X-rays were found to be normal, and he could say only that I didn't have arthritis. There were no bone, joint, or cartilage abnormalities. And if he had ordered fluid to be aspirated from the knee joint, the Lyme infection would still not have been identified. Like other specialists, he was trained to see symptoms in isolation, based on stringent norms, and therefore had nothing to offer. However, he scheduled another visit, and when I was, by that time, too sick to come, he called to find out how I was.

IN THE HOSPITAL

Just a couple of weeks later, I was admitted to the Metrowest Hospital in Framingham, where I spent five days feeling profoundly ill with a deep nausea. I lay in a hospital bed in a gown, propped against pillows and watching the nurses' station. It was morning and physicians milled around the desk, looking at medical records while murmuring softly to each other. I could hear their voices, so they must have been nearby, but they appeared to be far away. I didn't know where the entrance to the unit was, or what floor I was on. I was a distant observer, helpless and afraid.

I knew what my problem had to be, but why did no one else? Why the veil of silence after an ordinary backyard tick bite? Only the kindly white-haired neurologist who had admitted me recognized that I was even ill. He ordered tests, many tests, and a parade of specialists came and went by my bed. I told the infectious disease specialist that my knees hurt and that I had a tick bite and rash. Could this be Lyme? Oh no. He was adamant. But he ordered a Western blot test, which came back negative. While the Western blot test is a better test than the one I had been given previously, it, too, misses many cases.

I lay on my stomach on a table while a surgeon snipped a small piece of muscle from the back of my thigh. That test also was normal.

The nerve conduction test was normal. The rheumatologist at the Metrowest Hospital ascribed my swollen knees to lack of exercise. Still, the neurologist knew I was sick but was unable to identify the cause. Many diseases were ruled out, but the true diagnosis of Lyme disease could not be made.

When I was about to be sent home without a medical diagnosis, a psychiatrist came by my bed to recommend that I make an appointment with him after I left the hospital. He followed up by cornering my family in the hall. I ordered him out, undoubtedly making him all the more certain I needed his services. I told him I knew I had Lyme. He said, "If you don't like me, I can recommend someone else." The conversation ended. He sent no bill.

It is not uncommon for those with Lyme disease to be referred to psychologists or psychiatrists. The usual laboratory tests are negative. There is no diagnosis. Pain may not have physical signs. And if patients are ill, worried, frustrated, or angry, the opinion may be offered that "it's all in her head." Accepting this interpretation without question can result in seriously delayed treatment, leading to exacerbated illness and permanent disability.

STILL NO DIAGNOSIS

Physician education for Lyme disease is almost nonexistent. My physicians did not view Lyme disease as that serious, and in their minds, I had already been treated according to the only guidelines that they knew. If they had seen persistent Lyme disease cases before my case, they had not recognized them as such. During my search, physicians made occasional suggestions that I had chronic fatigue syndrome, or, because of the pain, fibromyalgia, meaning pain without known cause, disease categories characterized by unexplained, intense fatigue that is not relieved by sleep, and pain that may be transitory and occurs in one or many parts of the body. The causes of these ongoing, and often disabling conditions are unknown. There is speculation that they may be due to an autoimmune disorder or a virus, but increasingly, chronic fatigue syndrome and fibromyalgia are recognized as symptoms of Lyme disease.

The Arthritis Foundation lists Lyme disease as a possible cause of arthritis. I spoke to its medical consultant in Newton, Massachusetts, and he was as puzzled as all the rest. He knew nothing of persisting or chronic Lyme disease, or of treatment options. He could give no referrals to physicians who might have experience with Lyme disease that is not cured in a month. He gently steered me toward accepting fibromyalgia as a diagnosis. Arthritis and fibromyalgia, as well as chronic fatigue syndrome, are categories of disease with problematic and multiple meanings. Arthritis, or painful joints, can have many causes. Fibromyalgia and chronic fatigue syndrome are not fully understood and have no diagnostic tests. These conditions describe unexplained pain in the body and tiredness that goes beyond the experience of normal fatigue.

I made an appointment with a rheumatologist at the Newton-Wellesley Hospital, located in a Boston suburb. He listened carefully and seemed to accept my opinion that this might be Lyme, but when he learned that I'd had the problem for several months, he didn't understand. He didn't know about Lyme disease that lasted beyond a few weeks. He gave me a prescription for a sleep medication and said, "There's a very good fibromyalgia man at the Newton-Wellesley Hospital. It'll take you a few months to get an appointment, but he's very good. Here is his telephone number."

Others Have Lyme Disease

Later, after much research, I discovered that I was not alone with this illness. A fitness instructor at a gym, who has a large garden and several dogs, lay in bed on antibiotics for three months with Lyme disease. A man in the hospital for a month with intravenous antibiotics for Lyme disease entered a rehabilitation center to regain the use of his hands. A woman who said she felt tired and "achy," had painful knees and difficulty sleeping, was treated a year ago for Lyme disease.

Earlier, I had known two people with mysterious illnesses, one a weekend bicyclist and hiker who became ill with a numbing fatigue. Sometimes she lay on a foam mattress on her office floor in order to get through the workday. The other, following his retirement, had cleared brush and landscaped his home, gotten several tick bites, and become tired and dizzy. His many tests at the Massachusetts General Hospital gave no answers, and he was told only that it wasn't Lyme.

I learned that the Massachusetts Department of Public Health had a Lyme and tick-borne diseases task force that held meetings attended by state officials and physicians, and that the meetings were open to the public. While there I met other Lyme patients with long-term disease. With all due care for our health, attention to tick removal, and good health insurance, we found ourselves sitting around a rectangular table in large wooden chairs in the conference room of an aging state nursing school building in Canton, Massachusetts.

A mother of two said that both she and her two children have chronic Lyme disease. She was told, mistakenly, that she had multiple sclerosis. Bacteria had attacked the brain of one child resulting in a psychiatric hospitalization in a locked ward. Not believing their daughter's illness was psychological, her parents removed her from the institution and began their search for help. They found two published articles, Dr. Robert Bransfields's "Neuropsychiatric Assessment of Lyme Disease," and Dr. Brian Fallon's "Neuropsychiatric Manifestations of Lyme Borreliosis." Four months later their daughter was diagnosed with Lyme disease by Dr. Charles Ray Jones, a pediatric Lyme disease specialist in New Haven, Connecticut, and began her road to recovery.

A young woman with long black hair, recently married, with plans to be a dancer, got Lyme disease in a European forest at some time during her teen years. She attended Boston University using crutches. When she discovered at the university that the cause of her disability was Lyme disease, she went back to Europe to find the standard treatment there to be limited to six weeks. So she returned to the United States and was now finally receiving treatment for her disease.

Another woman had planned to spend the summer after college in Washington working on Capitol Hill, but her parents worried about her safety in the big city, so instead she went on a camping trip to Minnesota, a state with a high rate of Lyme disease. Since that trip twenty years ago, she has never been well. She said the swelling in her brain made it difficult for her to follow the discussion at the meeting that we had just attended. Her husband, at work in Boston that day, also has chronic Lyme disease.

A fourth woman at the meeting, after years of undiagnosed Lyme disease, lost her sight after it attacked her eyes. Over the years she had removed many ticks. After a life in the suburban outdoors with gardens, children, and dogs, and hours spent lying in the grass looking at clouds, she became ill with frequent unexplained sore throats and bouts of disabling fatigue. Nothing in the training or experience of her physician husband prepared him for the chronic disease that would plague his family.

This woman says she always felt she had an infectious disease. She saw a well-known infectious disease specialist in Boston who was certain that he would be able to help her. But when, at the end of a month of antibiotics she was no better, he dismissed her without understanding why she was sick. Several years later, at a Wellesley College reunion in 1989, she spoke to a graduate student in biology who suggested the possibility of Lyme disease as the cause of her illness. She and her doctor searched for all available information and consulted with a New York physician who treats chronic Lyme disease, and she learned that she had it.

THE TICKS THAT MAKE YOU SICK

I probably acquired my disease on Cape Cod when I bought additional land that surrounded my vacation house. It was November and I thought the tick season was over. I didn't know that ticks can become active if the outside temperature rises much above 35 degrees Fahrenheit. I wore boots over gray sweat pants, but they did not prevent the tick from crawling up to my waist and finding skin. But it is also possible that I acquired the disease at my suburban home in Wayland.

The tick was deeply burrowed under the skin on the back of my hip, and it was dried out, desiccated, the doctor said when he removed it. The bite had obviously occurred a long time ago, and the tick had not dropped off. Although the bite did not produce a rash until May when the tick was removed, the bug had probably been there about six months. After November, when I'd raked leaves around the bushes in my suburban yard, I was not outdoors amidst woods or fields until spring, and the tick was too dried out to have produced a recent bite. I had no pets that could have brought it into my house.

On that day in the meeting in Canton, Massachusetts, I met eight people with persisting or chronic Lyme disease. As the Lyme community organized and found its voice, I met men, women, and children, all with chronic disease.

Many cases of Lyme resolve in a few weeks. Sometimes heard is "I've had it three times." This occurs so regularly that the possibility of serious disability seldom becomes evident, either in news articles or doctors' offices. Others have ongoing illness with symptoms so mild that, as one woman says, "It could be Lyme disease but I can live with it." I was one of the 10 percent of those infected who became seriously ill.

If your disease is not cured in a few weeks, you may be told, mistakenly, that you have chronic fatigue syndrome, or that your excruciating pain is due to fibromyalgia, to an unknown virus, new allergies, or other chronic conditions that we don't yet know about. Lyme bacteria enter the brain, often within days, or even hours, of infection, with the result that, as the disease progresses, you may be told, also mistakenly, that you have multiple sclerosis or Parkinson's disease, or even Alzheimer's disease. Your children may have learning difficulties, arthritic pain, be unable to stay awake or participate in sports. They may have frequent infections and absences from school, when formerly they were active, successful students. Physicians from whom you seek answers are untrained in evaluating and treating ongoing Lyme disease, and they are usually frustrated and unable to help.

With undiagnosed illness, families can be torn apart. Chronic fatigue can make holding a job difficult or impossible, and medical insurance can be lost. Very often, spouses try to help but find it hard to remain understanding when their partners never seem to get well. Some children must be homeschooled. Marriages sometimes dissolve and parenting becomes difficult. My neighbor, diagnosed after many years, says, "I wanted to go to my sons' games and attend teacher conferences but I just couldn't." Thousands have found their ongoing illnesses to be Lyme and are receiving treatment for their long-undiagnosed disease.

The Lyme Controversy and Chronic Disease

While information on the nature of the disease is readily available, the story of the controversy remains largely untold. Physicians who are experienced in treating persisting disease have treated hundreds, or thousands, of cases similar to mine, and some have trod a rocky road, including loss of their medical licenses, for using clinical judgment instead of adhering to limitations published by the Infectious Diseases Society of America, a private, nonprofit, professional organization headquartered in Alexandria, Virginia.

There are two sides on the subject of chronic Lyme disease. We now know that, conservatively, 10 percent, and more likely 15 percent, of Lyme cases become chronic. The small group of fewer than a dozen physicians that determines policy for the IDSA, which includes Allen Steere, claims the disease is overdiagnosed and overtreated. This view can have significant consequences for those seeking timely medical care for Lyme disease.

Not all physicians limit diagnosis and treatment as recommended by that small policy-making group of physicians for the IDSA. There are those who no longer wait for rashes to appear. They give preventive antibiotics, and not just single doses, after a tick bite, as is frequently recommended. They learn from patients and from physicians who treat persistent Lyme disease. Many physicians now give six weeks or two months of antibiotic routinely and treat for several months if necessary. If relapse occurs, they treat their patients again. This is common sense. If this trend continues, we may see a reduction in the numbers of those with chronic disease.

You would expect that Lyme disease would be taken seriously, that every effort would be made to diagnose it early and treat it as completely as possible. But as you can see from my experience, and that of others, acknowledgment of the disease can be difficult or impossible, and finding adequate treatment is likely to be problematic for almost everyone who isn't cured in four weeks. Little has changed since I became ill in 1993, and in some ways the problem is worse, especially for those who are unaware of the politics of Lyme disease.

CONTROVERSIAL GUIDELINES

A major cause of the chronic Lyme disease problem has roots in events that occurred in 2000 that set the bar very high for diagnosing, and also for treating, Lyme disease. They advocate limiting treatment to a few weeks, regardless of how late the illness is diagnosed or how severe the illness, and fly in the face of much of what we know about the nature and persistence of Lyme bacteria. Lyme is a complex disease involving many strains of bacteria having characteristics that help them elude antibiotics. Nor are the guidelines substantiated by the clinical experience of physicians who treat serious Lyme disease.

Dr. Sam Donta was a member of the IDSA subcommittee while it was drafting the Lyme disease protocol. There was agreement only on the protocol for early disease. Donta wanted to add more information to the late-stage section, but others on the subcommittee disagreed. The science was not argued and, by this protocol, the existence of chronic Lyme disease was denied, and persisting symptoms became designated "post-Lyme syndrome." Donta refused to sign the document as drafted, and without his concurrence, his name was removed from the guidelines.

To this day, the writers of the guidelines have produced no evidence for the theory of "post-Lyme syndrome." Although admitting that continuing symptoms will occur in 10 to 20 percent of patients, they say that these may be due to an unexplained autoimmune reaction, and that continuing symptoms are no different from the pains people experience in their daily lives. Despite years of evidence and clinical experience that do not support the hypothesis, including testimony presented at state legislative hearings, they continue to resist the logical explanation, which is that symptomatic patients are still infected with Lyme bacteria. Therein lies the controversy and the problem for those who become victims of this disease.

Guidelines that were written for early disease then became the protocol for all Lyme disease, whether discovered early or late, guidelines that physicians have barely understood, and from which most have hardly dared deviate. While adherence to them is voluntary, they are heavily promoted and may be the only source of information available to doctors. Physicians' clinical judgment in treating patients was reduced or replaced by guidelines that became standard, and the only ones that most physicians know.

FINDING MEDICAL CARE

While many physicians use common sense and give treatment far beyond that recommended by the guidelines, others may be loath to use their clinical judgment to provide treatment that is adequate to prevent the disease from becoming chronic. As one patient reported:

> In August I had a tick bite and rash, although not a bull's-eye rash. I had two Lyme tests that were both negative, but my doctor gave me three weeks of doxycycline. I thought I was all right, but a few days later I got Bell's palsy, where

one side of my face drooped. Right after that, I got nerve pain in both arms; they burned and sometimes felt numb. Then the joints of one hand started to hurt and now I have pain. My legs began to hurt and lymph nodes swelled. I went back to my doctor and asked for more medicine because my symptoms were continuing to get worse. He said I didn't have Lyme. I didn't have a positive test. And if I did have Lyme, I didn't anymore because I was treated. I've had a CAT scan. They biopsied my lymph nodes because they thought I might have lymphoma. They thought it might be a virus. I've finally found a Lyme disease doctor, but he is so backed up I have to wait several months for an appointment. In the meantime, I have no treatment. I don't know what will happen if my disease is not treated soon. What can I say to persuade my primary doctor to treat me until I can get an appointment with the specialist?"

The impact of these guidelines on the public's access to medical care for Lyme disease is substantial. The IDSA is a private organization, but its guidelines are published on the U.S. Centers for Disease Control (CDC) website which is readily available to doctors and the public. The CDC website, by providing only one point of view, limits information available to physicians, and, importantly, the guidelines make it possible for insurance companies to deny or limit reimbursement for Lyme disease.

ILADS GUIDELINES

Few physicians yet know that there is another set of guidelines published by the International Lyme and Associated Diseases Society (ILADS), a multidisciplinary medical organization in Bethesda, Maryland, dedicated to the diagnosis and appropriate treatment of Lyme and other tick-borne diseases. The two-hundred-member organization provides a forum for health science professionals, and among its goals is improved physician understanding of Lyme disease and encouraging Lyme disease research on chronic disease. It is composed of physicians and healthcare providers who are experienced in treating chronic Lyme and other tick-borne diseases, and its guidelines are very different from those of the IDSA.

Because of unrealistic IDSA diagnostic guidelines making it harder for physicians to recognize this complex disease, delayed diagnosis can result in lack of timely treatment. This increases the risk that patients will not recover in four weeks. And because of restrictive treatment guidelines, many will not receive treatment beyond four weeks, when, with delayed diagnosis, they may need months or more, using combinations of antibiotics far more effective than the standard dose of the antibiotic doxycycline. Finding a physician who understands and treats persistent Lyme disease, who treats patients until they are well, remains a challenge for those whose disease is not easily cured.

On October 12, 2006, IDSA allowed its guidelines to be debated for the first time ever at the IDSA Conference in Toronto, Canada. Before an audience of five hundred, Dr. Paul Auerter, associate professor of Medicine at Johns Hopkins University, debated Dr. Raphael Stricker, president of the International Lyme and Associated Diseases Society. Although the IDSA has eight thousand members, only a few are involved in drafting guidelines that affect so many physicians and their patients. After the debate, some IDSA members expressed concern at turning away patients in order to follow guidelines.

The politics of Lyme disease continue to limit physician communication, trivialize a potentially serious disease, derail treatment, and politicize research. The near-inaccessibility of Lyme disease treatment remains virtually invisible. The refusal to accept the fact that a patient has Lyme disease allows treatment to be denied.

I have given you an overview of the problem. Knowing the controversy helps you avoid possible serious illness. Other infectious diseases have had their problems, as initial doubts are expressed, conflicting evidence is presented, and competing interests seek ascendancy. But while other diseases have had their politics, there has been nothing like what has occurred with Lyme disease.

CHAPTER TWO

"HAVE WE ALWAYS HAD LYME?"

DISCOVERING INFECTIOUS DISEASE, ENVIRONMENTAL CHANGE, AND THE SURGE OF LYME DISEASE

We came from China to the United States last year. Now we have Lyme disease. My children are very young and they are sick. The doctor says only my husband has Lyme disease and gave him two weeks of antibiotic. He will not give him any more. He will not give me and my children any antibiotic. I have fatigue and my muscles hurt. My knees hurt. It is hard to sleep. I have other things that are wrong, too. What shall I do?

—HARVARD GRADUATE STUDENT

Despite the surge in Lyme disease and increasing numbers of infected ticks, none of the four Lyme disease cases cited in the quote above will be counted in state health department statistics. The members of this family have been sick for at least five months and have become part of the hidden epidemic. Three of them don't meet the restrictive Infectious Diseases Society of America guidelines and have not been diagnosed by their doctor. Unlike other infectious diseases, such as eastern equine encephalitis (a viral disease spread by infected mosquitoes), meningitis, measles, or West Nile virus, the reporting of Lyme disease is not a high priority. Not only is the medical community divided on diagnosis and treatment of the disease, there is also the reporting problem that helps keep the Lyme epidemic hidden.

If people died from Lyme, as occurs with AIDS, the Lyme epidemic would not likely remain out of public view. Or if people became acutely ill immediately following a tick bite, as some do, the disease would be reported. If the symptoms were always consistent and visible to others, it would be acknowledged. And if Lyme were a contagious disease, passed from person to person, or acquired through contaminated food or water, in short, a public health problem, government and medicine would address it in a very different way.

No other infectious disease has had the controversy and politics that occurs with Lyme. It is a disease caused by bacteria that live in the landscape surrounding our houses with the potential to invade large areas of our bodies. It has an uncertain course and doubtful outcome. Those on both sides of the controversy, those who say the disease is overdiagnosed and overtreated and the others saying the disease should be treated until a person is well, accept that the number of infected people is at least ten times the reported number.

With many years of mounting evidence on persisting disease, it seems ironic that the IDSA and its supporters continue to flood professional journals and the media with messages that trivialize the potential impact of Lyme's disease on people's lives. For example, a *Forbes* magazine article stated, "The typical Lyme infection responds to simple antibiotics. Symptoms like arthritis and fatigue may linger in a subset of patients."[1] The results of articles such as this are not inconsequential. With this view that Lyme is not a serious disease, the public faces lack of medical care and insurance coverage for an unacknowledged and undiagnosed illness.

Discovering Other Infectious Diseases

Lyme is only one of many infectious diseases that afflict people. We know how it is transmitted, by deer ticks, and how it spreads through the body, by motile corkscrew-shaped bacteria. We have observed them under the microscope and have options for treating the disease, described in Chapter 8. We have information that would allow us to move forward in understanding this many-faceted illness. With the public remaining largely unprotected from the effects of this potentially devastating disease, there are questions that are always asked.

"Why are the science and clinical evidence ignored?
Has this happened with other infectious diseases?
Have we always had Lyme?
Why is it so prevalent now?"

These questions are answered in this and Chapter 3 on the discovery of Lyme disease.

For centuries, epidemics have swept through civilizations, with the causes unknown. Bacteria and viruses were as yet undiscovered. In early America, as records and gravestones show, life was uncertain, and even into the twentieth century, people sickened and died, often with little warning. The causes of death included pneumonia, smallpox, typhoid fever, tuberculosis, diphtheria, streptococcal infections, scarlet fever, and in southern regions of the country, yellow fever. Families were often large, but not every child was expected to live into adulthood. There seemed no way to prevent diseases and no way to treat them beyond so-called home remedies, such as herbs, poultices, and leeches. Medical remedies of earlier times often favored removing a disease by methods such as bleeding and purging, either with an enema or by blistering, or perhaps by using calomel, a form of mercury.

Sufferers could not always identify the illness that they had. They were said to be sick with "fever."

Although many scientists have acquired and provided the knowledge that has changed our lives, some have become icons in discovering and conquering infectious diseases, making possible the progress that has occurred in understanding their causes, transmission, and treatment. Among those scientists most well known in microbiology are Antony van Leeuwenhoek, Edward Jenner, Ignaz Semmelweiss, Louis Pasteur, Robert Koch, Joseph Lister, and Alexander Fleming. Their discoveries did not always lead to immediate acceptance. Throughout time, there have been disbelief and conflict with accepted theories of sickness and healing, but nothing comparable to the denial and conflict that we see today for Lyme disease.

The work of these seven scientists established the foundation for identifying other bacterial diseases, including Lyme. From their work came the development of powerful microscopes and visualization of microorganisms. They learned about bacteria and immunization against disease-causing organisms. Antiseptic surgical techniques were developed to prevent illness, and curative antibiotics were discovered.

Jenner's discovery of the smallpox vaccine was resisted initially, and for a long time it was available only to a privileged few, as was the earlier discovery of vaccination in Turkey. Semmelweiss's discovery of the need for physicians in obstetrics to wash their hands was opposed, even with supportive data, because fellow physicians did not consider unclean hands to be the cause of death in women whom they treated in their clinics. However, Louis Pasteur's discovery of the microorganisms affecting the wine and silk industries produced economic benefits and was accepted gladly. When he developed the anthrax vaccine, it provided immediate assistance to the cattle industry in France.

ANTONY VAN LEEUWENHOEK (1632–1723)

A tradesman in Delft, Holland, Antony van Leeuwenhoek, with no higher education or university degrees, would normally have been excluded from the scientific community of his time. Nevertheless, he made discoveries that opened the world of microscopic life to future scientists. In 1648 he saw his first microscope, a magnifying glass used by fabric merchants to examine cloth. Leeuwenhoek was also familiar with glassmaking and began to work with lenses. He experimented with grinding them and eventually built more than five hundred microscopes that were far superior to those of his day. As a businessman, he protected his method of building microscopes, fearing that the scientific world would disregard or forget his role in microscopy. Leeuwenhoek was the first to observe living microorganisms, and he made observations on what he saw. He examined bacteria, sperm cells, red blood cells, nematodes, or roundworms, and other forms of microscopic life that no one had ever seen before. In water to which he had added peppercorns, he observed after three weeks the sudden appearance of a number of "very little animals." And among his many experiments, he examined the plaque between his teeth and saw an "unbelievably great company of living animalcules." Thoughout his long life, he entertained visitors willingly, setting up displays so they could observe his specimens. Among the visitors who traveled to Delft were the tsar of Russia and the future James II of England.

Leeuwenhoek's career as tradesman and civic figure took a new turn in 1673 when a physician friend and anatomist in Delft introduced him by letter to the Secretary of the Royal Society of London, who encouraged him to begin a correspondence, even though Leeuwenhoek spoke only Dutch and his letters required translation. In 1676, some of his observations were met with skepticism by members of the society, so at Leeuwenhoek's insistence, the society sent an English vicar along with a team of respected jurists and doctors to Delft to determine whether he could observe and reason clearly. His observations were validated, and over the next fifty years Leeuwenhoek wrote more than three hundred letters to the Royal Society. He was elected a fellow in 1680, and after his death seven of his microscopes were donated to the Society.

Leeuwenhoek's observations were recorded in letters, not in scientific papers, that he wrote in conversational style to the society and to friends. In a 1715 letter he wrote,

> Some go to make money out of science, or to get a reputation in the learned world. But in lens-grinding and discovering things hidden from our sight, these count for naught . . . And I am satisfied too that not one man in a thousand is capable of such study, because it needs much time . . . and you must always keep thinking about these things if you are to get any results.

On June 12, 1716, he wrote:

> My work . . . was not pursued in order to gain the praise I now enjoy, but chiefly from a craving after knowledge, which I notice resides in me more than in most other men. And therewithal, whenever I found out anything remarkable, I have thought it my duty to put down my discovery on paper, so that all ingenious people might be informed thereof.

He opened a world that was hitherto unknown, and his work was not controversial because he described what he saw without interpretion. However interesting his observations, the connection was not made between Leeuwenhoek's early discoveries and infectious disease, and his work played no part in Jenner's later discovery of vaccination against smallpox.

EDWARD JENNER (1749–1823)

As an English country doctor practicing medicine in the town of Berkeley, Edward Jenner apprenticed with a local surgeon, followed by attendance at St. George's, University of London. In 1773, he returned to his hometown in the county of Gloucestershire to begin his medical practice. Jenner was a man of wide intellectual interests in science, medicine, and nature. From the beginning, he maintained his professional connections and started a society where physicians met to dine and read scientific papers. In his medical practice, he observed what others had noted, that dairymaids, after contracting cowpox, a less virulent and deadly disease that is related to smallpox, did not get smallpox. He knew about the Turkish practice of inoculation against smallpox, which was done by women, not by those in the world of medicine and science. The probable reason that this earlier discovery was not credited as first is that Jenner was the first in the Western world.

On May 14, 1796, he performed a historic experiment. A milkmaid named Sarah Nelmes visited him for treatment of cowpox. Jenner inoculated his gardener's eight-year-old son, James Phipps, with material from the pockmarks of the milkmaid. The boy contracted cowpox but recovered. Eight weeks later, Jenner completed his experiment by exposing him to smallpox, and the boy did not get the disease. The inoculation had protected him against smallpox.

Two years later, in 1798, after more successful cases, Jenner wrote his book, *An Inquiry Into the Causes and Effects of the Variolae Vaccine*. The medical community initially rejected his claims, and he responded by donating free vaccine to hospitals. Later, a similar experiment in London with cowpox and smallpox validated his work. The serum was hard to obtain and keep preserved, and inoculation methods used by other doctors varied, but the number of smallpox deaths decreased. If people became ill, they were far less sick if they had been vaccinated. Jenner named his procedure *vaccination* (*vacca* is the Latin word for "cow").

In 1811 he moved to London and in 1813 was awarded the MD degree. In later life, he received many honors and was rewarded for the development of the vaccine and for his continuing research. The home and small hut in his garden where he performed his vaccinations have been preserved. Jenner is known as the "father of infectious disease study"; his discovery of prevention paved the way not only for the eradication of a deadly illness but also for the development of modern immunology.

Many years before Jenner's work, Lady Mary Wortley Montagu (1689–1762) made a major contribution to acceptance of Jenner's discovery in 1796. As wife of the English ambassador, she arrived in Turkey in 1719. As recorded in her prolific writings, she immersed herself in all aspects of the country's customs, including learning to speak the Turkish language. During extensive travels, she became acquainted with upper-class women who knew about inoculation. Her brother had died of smallpox, and Lady Mary's face was scarred as a result of the disease. While in Turkey, she had her infant son vaccinated. She describes the inoculation process in a letter to her friend, Sarah Chiswell.

> People send to one another to know if any of their family has a mind to have the small-pox [*sic*] they make parties for this purpose, and when they are met (commonly fifteen or sixteen together) the old woman comes with a nut-shell full of the matter of the best sort of small-pox [*sic*] and asks what vein you please to have opened. She immediately rips open the vein that you offer to her with a large needle (which gives you no more pain than a common scratch) and puts into a vein as much matter [substance from the pustules] as can lie easily on the head of her needle, and after that, binds up the little wound with a hollow bit of shell, and in this manner opens four or five veins . . . The children or young patients play together the rest of the day, and are in perfect health until the eighth. Then the fever begins to seize them, and they keep their beds [*sic*] two days, very seldom three. They have very rarely above twenty or thirty [pustules] on their faces, which never mark, and in eight days time they are as well as before their illness. . . . Where they are wounded there

34

remains running sores during the distemper, which I
don't doubt is a great relief to it.[2]

Montagu wrote that the French ambassador told her that every year
thousands were inoculated, that they "took the small-pox" as they did
"the waters" in other countries, and that no one had ever died from it.
She says in her letter:

> I am patriot enough to bring this useful invention into
> fashion in England, and I should not fail to write to some
> of our doctors very particularly about it, if I knew any one
> of 'em that I thought had virtue enough to destroy such
> a considerable branch of their revenue for the good of
> mankind, but that distemper is too beneficial to them not
> to expose to all their resentment the hardy wight [sic] that
> should undertake to put an end to it.

Lady Mary did indeed bring her discovery back to England, where
her daughter was also inoculated. She introduced the practice to the
English nobility, and although some were inoculated, there was, as she
had predicted, medical and religious opposition, which, for a variety
of reasons, lasted well into the nineteenth century. Vaccination, however, was not available to the general public. In France, Voltaire, a proponent of vaccination, convinced Catherine the Great of Russia to be
vaccinated, and her entire court was inoculated against smallpox.

As a result of Lady Mary's discovery in Turkey, the practice of inoculation was introduced into the United States by the physician Zabdiel
Boylston of Boston. The Puritan minister Cotton Mather supported
the practice. He had learned of it from a slave who had been inoculated in Africa, and he encouraged Boylston to try it. As a result, Boylston inoculated his only son and two slaves, all of whom recovered in
about a week. But opposition was strong. Opponents feared that vaccination would spread the disease, and some even urged that Boylston

be tried for murder. George Washington and Benjamin Franklin were strong proponents of vaccination to help control outbreaks of small-pox, and in Virginia, Thomas Jefferson had eighteen of his relatives vaccinated.

The substance used for the inoculation, including the amount, was not standardized, and people could become ill for days or weeks. During the 1764 smallpox epidemic in Boston, thirty years before Jenner's discovery, John Adams describes his experience with inoculation, speaking of the "lancet dividing the skin," into which an "infected thread" was laid in the "channell" [*sic*]. Adams and his brother, along with nine other patients, were confined to the hospital for three weeks with aches, pains, fever, and eruption of pockmarks. Eleven years after John Adams was inoculated, in 1775, Abigail Adams, wrote in one of her many letters to her husband that because of an outbreak of smallpox, she brought her children to Boston for vaccination. One of them became quite ill and the family stayed in Boston for two months. But until the mid-nineteenth century, the number of those inoculated was low.

From 1885 to 1945, vaccines were developed for other diseases, including rabies, cholera, typhoid, diphtheria, pertussis (whooping cough), tuberculosis, tetanus, and yellow fever. The first influenza (flu) vaccines were used in 1945. In 1963 the measles vaccine was licensed, and the rubella (German measles) vaccine was licensed two years later.

Despite discoveries in immunization, the causes of infectious diseases were still unknown. Bacteria were not discovered until much later, not until near the end of the nineteenth century. And although some diseases could be prevented or mitigated by inoculation, many others could not, but might instead be prevented by environmental sanitation, as was discovered by Ignaz Semmelweiss.

IGNAZ SEMMELWEISS (1818–1865)

Known as the famed physician who introduced hand washing as a way to prevent disease, Ignaz Semmelweiss discovered the cause of puerperal fever, commonly known as childbed or childbirth fever. He did not know about bacteria but concluded that the cause of infectious disease was a particle of some sort that was transmitted from one person to another. As many as a quarter of previously healthy women died in hospitals from infection in the nineteenth century. During the seventeenth century, hospitals for childbirth were developed in several major European cities, serving as training facilities for doctors. They were crowded, and doctors performed many examinations. They used instruments regularly, allowing wide opportunity for infection to spread from contaminated instruments as well as dressings and bedding. During the eighteenth century, hospitals in Europe and America consistently reported deaths from 20 to 25 percent in childbirth wards, and it was even said that during epidemics, the number could be 100 percent. The first recorded epidemic of childbed fever occurred in Paris in 1646.

Others before Semmelweiss had considered that the disease was spread by medical practitioners. In 1795, Alexander Gordon in Scotland suggested that childbirth fever was the result of an infectious process, and in 1842 in England Thomas Watson wrote that wherever puerperal fever was prelevant, the practitioner should use "most diligent ablution."

In 1843, Oliver Wendell Holmes in Boston published his well-known treatise, "The Contagiousness of Puerperal Fever" and suggested that the disease was spread to patients by their doctors. After graduating from Harvard College, Holmes pursued his medical studies in the Parisian hospital system and then returned to Harvard, where he received his medical degree. Later, he became professor of anatomy and physiology there.

Holmes recommended hand washing, clean clothing, and the avoidance of autopsies by those aiding birth. He said, ". . . in my own family, I had rather that those I esteemed the most should be delivered unaided in a stable . . . than that they should receive the best help in the fairest apartment, but exposed to the vapors of this pitiless disease." Holmes's conclusions were ridiculed by many contemporaries, including the prominent obstetrician Charles Meigs, who made his well-known statement, "Doctors are gentlemen, and gentlemen's hands are clean."

In Vienna, Semmelweiss was unaware of Holmes's treatise. After he graduated from the Second Vienna Medical School, he remained for a course in midwifery and a master's degree. After completing his surgical training, he spent fifteen months learning diagnostic and statistical methods. In 1846 he became obstetrical assistant in the First Obstetrical Clinic of the Vienna General Hospital, considered to be the best hospital in Vienna. At the time, puerperal fever killed 13.1 percent of women who entered that hospital, and it was said that many women preferred to give birth in the streets rather than go to that hospital. In the Second Obstetrical Clinic, however, the death rate was only 2.0 percent. Both clinics were in the same hospital, the only difference being that the first clinic was the teaching service for medical students, and the second clinic had been selected for the instruction of midwives.

In both hospital clinics, medical students did autopsies routinely. After a friend of Semmelweiss died after puncturing himself with a knife while doing an autopsy, at his friend's autopsy, Semmelweiss noted that the condition of the tissues appeared similar to that of women who had died of puerperal fever and hypothesized that particles from the cadavers were carried by hand to patients whom the students subsequently examined. Therefore, he instituted a policy of hand washing with chloride of lime after doing autopsies and before examining women. The death rate in the medical students clinic dropped from 12.24 percent at the beginning of the study to 2.38 percent, similar to that of the clinic staffed by midwives. During 1848 Semmelweiss went further in improving sanitation and ordered the washing of all instruments that came into contact with patients. With this, childbed fever was virtually eliminated from that hospital.

His findings went against the current scientific opinion that the disease was not preventable. A common view was that the disease resulted from imbalance of the basic "four humours" in the body. In addition, the washing of hands before seeing pregnant patients was too much work. Complaints were made that no scientific basis supported his theory, which is the same argument made today that says there is no evidence that Lyme disease can become chronic. Doctors did not want to accept that they might, unknowingly, have caused so many deaths. As for Lyme disease, the argument might be made that the IDSA's acceptance of persisting infection and need for continuing antibiotic treatment could open a Pandora's box for thousands of patients over the course of many years for whom medical care was denied.

For reasons unknown, Semmelweiss resisted presenting his findings to authorities in Vienna, and in 1849, partly because of national politics that became increasingly conservative, his contract was not renewed. When he left Vienna, the hand-washing and instrument-cleaning routines that he had introduced were eliminated, and once again, the number of deaths rose. In 1850, the year after Semmelweiss left, 35 out of 101 patients died, but even with those statistics and the shocking rise in maternal deaths, his theory was not accepted. Doctors returned to their old ways. From 1851 to 1857 Semmelweiss took charge of a maternity ward in Hungary, where his theory was put into practice, and the maternal mortality rate dropped to 0.85 percent. In 1857, he was offered a chair in obstetrics in Zurich but turned it down. He had a mental breakdown and died shortly thereafter.

Jenner and Semmelweiss, like others who made discoveries, had to take a proactive stand to move research forward. Semmelweiss took a position that challenged established medical practice, in effect charging physicians with procedures potentially harmful to their patients.

Those serving patient needs and treating chronic Lyme disease are challenging the position that too many antibiotics are used, and that antibiotics are unnecessary and even harmful. By doing this, some physicians have faced investigation by their medical boards and even lost their licenses to practice medicine.

In the United States, maternity hospitals continued to have outbreaks of puerperal fever until the discovery of antibiotics in the mid-twentieth century. Entire hospital wings could be shut down in order to contain the staphylococcus infection. The cause was known, but antibiotics were not yet available. They came into use during the late 1940s and early 1950s. Some of the restrictive hospital practices, such as isolating infants in nurseries and denying parents access to them, were based on fear of these outbreaks. At the same time, crowded conditions and multiple staff members, in varying conditions of health, who were caring for large numbers of women and babies, helped promote the spread of "staph" infections. These were the same infections that Semmelweiss had addressed almost a hundred years earlier by attempting to get physicians to wash their hands to reduce deaths in maternity wards.

LOUIS PASTEUR (1822–1895)

The germ theory of disease is the foundation of modern medicine. Although microorganisms had been seen by Leeuwenhoek, and hypothesized by Semmelweiss, it was the French scientist Louis Pasteur who discovered that they were the cause of infectious diseases. Pasteur believed in the freedom of creative imagination and rigorous experimentation and never hesitated to take issue with prevailing, yet false ideas of his time. He gave importance to the spread of knowledge and the application of research to benefit people's lives. He was a chemist, educated in Paris, and he spent several years teaching and doing research at Dijon and Strasbourg. In 1854 he became professor of chemistry at the University of Lille.

Pasteur's study of fermentation enabled him to understand changes that occur when wine ferments, milk turns sour, and meat decays. The souring of wine and beer was a major economic problem in France. When Pasteur examined sample droplets of bad beer under the microscope, he observed that it contained rod-shaped microorganisms instead of round yeast cells. Fermentation results from the action of a specific living microorganism, and Pasteur discovered how to culture those that are required to make good beer. He showed those in the wine industry that if wine is heated to 60 degrees (centigrade), the growth of harmful bacteria is prevented. He extended the discovery to milk by heating it to a higher temperature and pressure before bottling it, and the procedure became known as *pasteurization*.

Silkworm diseases were crippling the silk industry in France. In 1865, Pasteur discovered the microorganisms that caused the diseases and found that they were transmitted by an organism infesting the silkworms and spreading among them. He learned that they were also transmitted by heredity. Bacteria could multiply. As a result, the long-held theory that infectious agents arose from spontaneous generation was shown to be false. Diseases were not the result of bad air or "poisonous vapors," or "miasma," as they had been labeled since the Middle Ages.

Pasteur discovered that each disease was caused by a specific microbe, and that these foreign elements were not part of an organism. He observed, too, that some were anaerobic, living without oxygen, and with this discovery, he opened the door for the study of bacteria that cause septicemia and gangrene.

Large numbers of cattle in France were infected with anthrax, and outbreaks occurred over many years. In a major outbreak in the 1870s, many animals died. Some cows developed a more serious version of the illness than did others. With the expectation that they would die, Pasteur injected two cows with a strong dose of anthrax bacteria, and to his surprise, neither developed the disease. When he found that they had previously had the illness, he suspected they were immune to it and hypothesized that if it were possible to give an animal a mild attack of the disease, it would not contract the disease later on. He discovered the rod-shaped bacteria that cause anthrax and succeeded in developing a weakened and harmless culture, using it on cattle and sheep, and thereby solved a major problem for the cattle industry.

Pasteur is especially renowned for developing the rabies vaccine. Rabies is a highly infectious disease that attacks the nervous system. It results from the bite of a diseased animal or through infected saliva entering an existing wound. Pasteur injected an extract from the spinal column of a rabid dog into healthy animals, producing symptoms of rabies. After many attempts, Pasteur was able to develop a weakened, or attenuated, form of the virus that could be used for inoculation.

The vaccine had been tested on only eleven dogs before it was first used on a person. On July 6, 1885, after consulting with colleagues, Pasteur tested the vaccine on a nine-year-old boy, Joseph Meister, who had been bitten by a rabid dog. Without the vaccine, he faced almost certain death. Pasteur was not a licensed physician and could have faced prosecution. The boy recovered, and the success of the inoculation was heralded as an important discovery that aided the development of vaccines for other diseases. Pasteur, who received the highest honors of France, founded the Pasteur Institute, which still exists in Paris as an important center for the study of infectious diseases.

ROBERT KOCH (1843–1910)

The two scientists recognized as being the principle figures in the development of the science of bacteriology are Louis Pasteur and Robert Koch. It was Koch who learned the bacterial cause of tuberculosis. Tuberculosis has existed since antiquity, as we know from the study of ancient tubercular bones. Often known as "consumption," it could be a lingering, and often fatal, illness, which afflicted rich and poor alike. During the nineteenth century, one in seven European deaths was ascribed to the disease.

After graduating from the University of Gottingen in Germany in 1866, Robert Koch served in the Franco-Prussian War, then later became a district medical officer in Wollstein. He discovered that apparently spontaneous outbreaks of anthrax in cattle were, in fact, due to long-living endospores (a dormant form of the bacteria allowing them to survive for long periods under harsh conditions) that were embedded in the soil. As a result, he was rewarded with a job at the Imperial Health Office in Berlin.

In Berlin, as during much of his career, the laboratory facilities were minimal and his work was done in cramped spaces. Nevertheless, he improved his laboratory techniques of purification, staining, and bacterial growth media, including agar plates (a gelatinous substance used as a culture medium for growing microorganisms) and the petri dish, both still used today. With these techniques, he discovered the mycobacterium tuberculosis. Koch continued studying infectious diseases, including cholera, and in 1883 was sent to Egypt as leader of the German Cholera Commission. He brought back pure cultures and continued his studies of cholera in India.

Koch formulated rules, or postulates, for the control of epidemics that were approved by the Great Powers (Great Britain, France, Germany, Russia, Austria-Hungary, and Italy) in Dresden in 1893 and are still in use. He said that to establish that an organism is the cause of disease, it must be (1) found in all cases of the disease examined, (2) prepared and maintained in a pure culture, (3) capable of producing an original infection, even after several generations in culture, and (4) retrievable from an inoculated animal and cultured again.

For Lyme disease, these conditions pose a problem because we can't easily find the causative bacteria in the body, and the microorganism can be grown only in a very specific culture. It replicates slowly, dividing approximately once every twenty-four hours in comparison to other organisms that may divide in minutes. Retrieval from an inoculated animal is difficult or impossible, although bacteria may sometimes be detected in the rash.

JOSEPH LISTER (1827–1912)

Listerine® mouthwash was named for Joseph Lister, an English surgeon who, after attending the University of London, obtained a professorship at the University of Glasgow. Lister introduced antiseptic techniques into hospitals to prevent infectious disease. The common explanation for wound infection at the time was that exposed tissues were damaged by chemicals in the air. The surgical wards smelled because of rotting wounds, and only occasionally were they aired out. There were no facilities for washing hands before cleaning patients' wounds.

Between 1861 and 1865, in the male ward of the Glasgow Royal Infirmary, between 45 and 50 percent of the amputation cases died from infection. While working at the infirmary, Lister learned of the work of Louis Pasteur, who had demonstrated that if microorganisms were present, rotting and fermentation could occur without oxygen because of the presence of anaerobic bacteria. Lister confirmed this finding with his own experiments.

Pasteur had recommended three methods of eliminating these anaerobic microorganisms: filtering them, heating them, or exposing them to chemical solutions. For human wounds, only the third method could be used. Therefore, Lister introduced the use of a 5 percent solution of carbolic acid, the older term for *phenol*, a colorless, slightly acidic toxic compound with antiseptic properties. It irritates the skin and was the reason surgical gloves were first introduced. Its use markedly reduced the incidence of gangrene. Lister also required surgeons to wash their hands and wear clean gloves, and surgical instruments were sterilized. In 1867, he published a series of articles in *The Lancet* on "The Antiseptic Principle of the Practice of Surgery." Lister credited the earlier work of Semmelweiss on childbed fever as well, saying, "Without Semmelweiss, my achievements would be nothing." In 1869, he returned to the University of Edinburgh to continue his work on improving methods of sterilization.

DISCOVERING VIRUSES

Bacteria are one-celled organisms that do not contain a nucleus, as do human cells, and their shape ranges from spheres to rods to spirals. They live in every habitat on earth, including acidic hot springs and radioactive waste. They are only one type of infection-causing microorganism. Viruses are another type of infectious agent that, unlike bacteria, require living cells for replication and, until microscopes were improved, were too small to see. They cannot reproduce on their own and require a host cell to replicate. They cannot be killed with antibiotics, although we now have a few antiviral agents. Some viral diseases, such as rabies, can be prevented with vaccines.

The existence of infectious agents smaller than bacteria was suspected in the late nineteenth century. The Russian botanist Dimitri Iwanowski discovered that the sap of tobacco plants was infected with mosaic disease, even after being passed through a filter that would retain bacteria, and that the sap could infect healthy plants. In 1900, a similar result was obtained with foot-and-mouth disease in cattle. In 1935 in the United States, Wendell Meredith Stanley in the United States crystallized the tobacco mosaic virus and was awarded the 1946 Nobel Prize in Chemistry, which he shared with John Northrup and James Sumner.

In a chance meeting at an airport, Stanley met the president of the University of California at Berkeley, who was searching for a scientist to head the new biochemistry department, and, among other things, the two discussed the need for building a separate virus laboratory. As a result, in 1948, Stanley moved to Berkeley, staffing both the biochemistry department and the new virus laboratory that was funded by the California state legislature. While he was working at the laboratory, Stanley's interests and those of his staff turned to human and animal pathogens as well as those of plants. He studied poliomyelitis and developed an influenza vaccine. In later years, his interest turned to tumor-producing viruses in chickens.

Treatment for infectious diseases continued to remain elusive until well into the twentieth century. Disease-causing organisms were identified and immunization against some of them became possible. And the incidence could be reduced by sanitizing the environment. But what about treatment? How could infectious diseases be cured?

Today, we have some of the same curative issues with such chronic diseases as multiple sclerosis, Alzheimer's disease, and Parkinson's disease. Unlike with Lyme, a disease for which we know the cause, a great deal of medical attention is focused on these diseases. Though they are described in great detail, including their onset and symptoms, results of tests, and the courses they take, there is also the hard fact that for these diseases, available treatment options are limited, and there is, as yet, no cure. But with the discovery of antibiotics in the mid-twentieth century, it became possible to obtain truly miraculous cures for infectious diseases. The world of medicine was forever changed because of an accidental discovery of Sir Alexander Fleming.

ALEXANDER FLEMING (1881–1955)

Alexander Fleming, whose work made possible the treatment of infectious diseases, saw many soldiers die during World War I from infected wounds. Antiseptics that were used to disinfect their wounds were actually killing the soldiers by causing injury to body tissues and to the body's own defenses. Army physicians, however, continued to use them, even when the soldiers' conditions worsened. In addition, these antiseptics did not reach the anaerobic bacteria that continued to grow deep inside wounds, causing gangrene and tetanus.

Fleming was born on a remote sheep farm in northern Scotland, the seventh of eight children. After four years in a shipping office, he followed the career path of an older brother who was a physician and enrolled in St. Mary's Hospital in London to study medicine. He did not pursue his studies to become a surgeon but, instead, became a bacteriologist. After serving in World War I as a captain in the Army Medical Corps and working in battlefield hospitals at the Western Front in France, he returned to St. Mary's Hospital, which was a teaching hospital, and in 1928 became professor of bacteriology.

He was seeking antibacterial substances that would treat infection without harming human tissue. In his laboratory, while studying bacteria, he left agar plates containing bacterial cultures, sometimes for weeks, and observed what occurred. He noted that when mucous material from his nose was placed on an agar plate in a petri dish containing bacteria, the bacteria grew in abundance, except in the area surrounding the mucous sample, where the plate remained clear. He had discovered lysozyme, known as "the body's own antibiotic," which is found in some body secretions, including human tears, and published his findings in 1922.[3]

In 1928, while investigating staphylococcus bacteria, Fleming noted that many of his culture dishes were contaminated with a fungus and threw them into disinfectant. One day he was showing a visitor his work and retrieved one of the unsubmerged culture dishes. He noticed an area around the fungus where bacteria did not grow and concluded that the mold had, like lysozyme, created a bacteria-free zone around it. Fleming then isolated an extract from the mold and named the substance penicillin. He investigated its antibacterial effect on many organisms and found a positive effect on scarlet fever, pneumonia, gonorrhea, meningitis, and diphtheria. His discovery was published in 1929 in the *British Journal of Experimental Pathology*, but at that time the account of his findings received little attention.

Fleming found it difficult to cultivate the mold and to isolate the antibiotic agent, and many clinical tests were inconclusive. He continued until 1940 to try to interest a chemist in refining penicillin. In the early 1940s, penicillin was isolated and concentrated by Ernst Chain, but it required a team of scientists to produce a usable, purified, stable form of the antibiotic. In 1945, three researchers (Howard Florey, Ernest Chain, and Fleming) received the Nobel Prize, and Fleming was knighted for the discovery.

During his many lectures around the world, Fleming cautioned his listeners not to use penicillin unless there was a properly diagnosed reason, in order to avoid antibiotic resistance, and that when it was used, to never use too little or to use it for too short a period of time.

After Fleming's discovery, more antibiotics continued to be developed. Antibiotics, effective against bacteria, are drugs that either kill bacteria (bacteriocidal) or prevent the growth of bacteria (bacterio-static). If bacteriostatic drugs are used in sufficient quantity, they may also become bacteriocidal. Antibiotics are part of a class of drugs that are known as antimicrobials, and because antibiotics are relatively harmless to people, they can be used to treat infections. They are in-effective, however, against viral, fungal, or parasitic infections. The structures of viruses and fungi presented many more difficulties than were encountered with bacteria, and only many years later were an-tifungal and antiviral drugs introduced with any degree of success.

We now have a range of antibiotics to treat bacterial diseases. Some are broad spectrum, and effective against a large number of bacteria, while others target specific infections. Some diseases require multiple antibiotics. Although the principles of antibiotic action were not dis-covered until the twentieth century, more than 2500 years ago in China, molds such as those from soybean curd are reported to have been used. Plants were used to treat diseases, but the effective components were not identified and substances could not be purified.

With the foregoing developments in preventing and treating in-fectious diseases, it seemed that the scourge of infectious diseases might be at an end in the developed world. By the 1950s, penicillin became generally available for treating infectious diseases. "Strep throat," if treated in time, no longer resulted in rheumatic fever when streptococcal bacteria traveled to the heart. Bacteria-caused pneumo-nia could be cured, avoiding weeks and months of sickness. Within a few years, tuberculosis could be cured by using a combination of long-term antibiotics. Syphilis could be treated. Even Hansen's dis-ease (leprosy), dating from biblical times, could be treated by using long-term antibiotics.

Immunization against smallpox was so successful in eliminating the disease that vaccinations were discontinued in the United States in 1972. The last known case of smallpox occurred in Somalia in 1979, and in 1980, the World Health Organization declared smallpox eradicated from the world. In 2002, though, with fears of bioterrorism, some of the smallpox vaccine was brought out of storage.

With the introduction of the Salk polio vaccine in 1954, death and disability from "infantile paralysis" were eliminated in the United States. Vaccines for scarlet fever, pertussis ("whooping cough"), measles, and diphtheria became part of routine medical care, and quarantine signs were no longer posted on front doors of the sick. County tuberculosis sanatoriums were no longer needed and were closed.

Disease-causing organisms may be spread in a number of ways. Some viruses and bacteria are spread from person to person, by direct contact. Others are transmitted from animals to people, or from a mother to an unborn child. Microorganisms may be spread by droplet transmission through the air by coughs and sneezes. They can be transmitted to large numbers of people through contaminated food or water. Others, spread by rats, fleas, mosquitoes, or ticks, are known as vector-borne diseases. Lyme is a vector-borne disease.

The mosquito is the vector that carries yellow fever, the viral disease that decimated workers who built the Panama Canal. In the United States, yellow fever epidemics originated in port cities such as Philadelphia, where ships brought infected mosquitoes from the Orient. Typhus, carried by ticks and lice, remains common in many parts of the world. Rats carried infected fleas that spread the bubonic plague, known as the Black Death, across Asia and Europe in the fourteenth-century, wiping out a third of Europe's population.

Lyme Disease and Environmental Change

The vector that carries Lyme disease is the deer tick, which becomes infected with the disease by biting an already infected animal, usually either a mouse or a deer, and then injecting infected saliva into people when it seeks a blood meal. Deer ticks also carry diseases like Rocky Mountain spotted fever, tularemia, babesiosis, ehrlichiosis, anaplasmosis, bartonella, and others that continue to be identified.

Lyme-carrying ticks in the United States may be infected with any one of a hundred or more strains of Lyme bacteria, all having varying degrees of virulence, or the ability of the microbe to cause disease. "Virulence" derives from a Latin word meaning "full of poison."

Although experimental programs are being introduced, elimination of the tick is not possible, nor is it feasible to eliminate the increasing numbers of mice and deer that are associated with Lyme disease. With the loss of natural predators, such as the wolves, foxes, and coyotes that formerly controlled deer and mice populations, and with warmer climates that encourage the tick population growth, and with habitat change, the risk of people being bitten continues to increase. Every year we have more ticks, more infected ticks, and more Lyme disease occurring in more areas of the country. Other small animals besides mice carry Lyme disease. And there is an expanding human population moving into suburbs and coexisting with the escalating deer population.

Deer travel long distances, carrying their ticks wherever they go. A single deer may harbor dozens, and more, of small ticks, many of them on the neck and ears. Birds may also carry them long distances. When infected ticks bite deer, the deer become continuing infected reservoirs for Lyme disease but, for reasons unknown, do not become ill, as do horses, dogs, and other animals. They continue to carry the bacteria from infected ticks, and when uninfected ticks seek a blood meal, they become infected by the deer on which they feed. The white-footed mouse also becomes a reservoir for Lyme disease without becoming ill. When young ticks take their first blood meal from an infected mouse they become infected. When they take their second blood meal from a deer, they will then infect the deer if it hasn't already been. In turn, that deer infects all future ticks that take a blood meal. It's a vicious cycle.

Without the biodiversity of earlier times, we have exploding populations of mice, deer, and ticks, all associated with Lyme, and all with few or no natural enemies, living in an ever-shrinking habitat, and ever closer to the human population. Large numbers of oak trees contribute to the huge increase of deer, mice, and ticks. Oak leaf litter provides a haven for mice and ticks, and acorns are a favorite food source for deer and mice. Mark Jerome Walters describes the effect of habitat on emerging diseases.[4] The destruction and fragmentation of old-growth forests enable the spread of Lyme disease. When regrowth occurs, the woods are no longer the canopied parklike forests of old but are full of brush. Many species of plants and animals may not survive climate change, human incursion, and fragmented habitat that is crisscrossed with roads. Animals associated with proliferating Lyme disease, however, are unaffected by these factors. In fact, they thrive on them.

Deer survive well in fragmented forests with patches of light that encourage the growth of brush and succulent foliage they prefer. The brush makes them less visible to predators, and with fragmented forests, predators needing large hunting areas are less able to survive. Ticks are not found on higher tree branches of canopied forests that contain bushes. They follow the deer and prefer low-lying brush, shrubs, plants, and long grass. Mice live in all environments.

In more populated areas, mice and ticks like stone walls and woodpiles in suburban yards. Besides being attracted to edges of forests, deer also like yards where there are many plants they feed on. Ticks are commonly found along the borders of suburban yards, where they attach to brush and long grass, waiting for a blood meal. In small plots of land, ticks more readily find a human blood meal. Most tick bites are thought to occur in a yard where mice, deer, ticks, and humans live in close proximity.

Despite the increasingly favorable environmental conditions for it, Lyme disease was not recognized until 1975. By then, public health focus had turned to noninfectious diseases such as heart disease, diabetes, and cancer. When it was identified in Connecticut, the prevailing view was that infectious diseases had been largely controlled in developed countries, and there was a high degree of complacency toward them: We had antibiotics for infections. The public was warned to beware of ticks, but Lyme disease was not viewed as a major threat to public health.

Risks of a Lyme infection can be a major cause of disabling illness in our daily lives. Its discovery occurred in the time period after fears of infectious diseases had subsided, and before the resurgence of new infectious diseases. The next chapter tells the story of how Lyme, not a new disease, came to be discovered in America.

CHAPTER THREE

DISCOVERING LYME DISEASE

What does it take to get a disease discovered? How many cases of childhood arthritis would have been needed for Lyme to be recognized if not for Polly Murray's concern as a parent?

—MOTHER OF TWO CHILDREN WITH GESTATIONAL LYME DISEASE

Lyme was identified at a time of relative calm in regard to infectious diseases. When it came to the public's attention in 1975, it was viewed as an apparently new illness. Not until six years later, when the causative organism was identified, was it found to be an infectious disease whose symptoms can be arthritic, neurological, behavioral, cardiac, dermatological, muscular, or otherwise. The connection between ticks, bacteria, and rashes was not immediately evident.

During the 1970s on Long Island, a mysterious form of arthritis was dubbed "Montauk knee," for the town on its tip. Cases of Montauk knee, reported among fishermen and farmers since the 1960s, were later recognized as Lyme disease. However, during earlier days, when it was first reported, the connection between an insect bite and arthritis was not made. On nearby Shelter Island, Dr. Edgar Grunwaldt was using penicillin to treat what he saw as insect bites that caused an unusual rash.

Polly Murray initiated the process of identifying the disease that was crippling children in Lyme, Connecticut. Almost from the time they moved from New York City to their new home in the semirural town of Lyme, in the 1960s, Murray's family suffered from a variety of illnesses, the symptoms of which included rashes, painful and swollen joints, swollen glands, and neurological problems, which waxed and waned and became progressively worse. Doctors could not help them, and most of the physicians whom Murray saw considered her to be a hypochondriac.

By 1975, Murray knew what seemed an unusual number of children who had been diagnosed with juvenile rheumatoid arthritis, many of whom were on crutches, including her own children. More common in adults, it would have been less likely to come to her attention if not for the number of children affected—very much out of the ordinary. Without Murray's persistence, the disease might have remained unrecognized well beyond 1975.

Polly Murray called the Connecticut Department of Public Health and was told that arthritis is not a communicable or reportable disease, and therefore there was nothing the department could do. At about the same time, Judith Mensch in a neighboring town, who did not know Murray, independently called the department of public health, as well as the U.S. Centers for Disease Control. Mensch learned that the CDC had a program in which young doctors were assigned for epidemiological training to study locations and incidence of disease. One of these physicians, Dr. David Snydman, assigned to the Connecticut Department of Public Health, got in touch with Murray and Mensch. Snydman knew Allen Steere, who had also worked in the CDC program and had begun his career in rheumatology at Yale University. Snydman telephoned Steere.

Murray describes her first trip to Yale, a visit that lasted three hours, in her book, *The Widening Circle*.[1] She brought with her to Yale the stories of thirty-five people with problems similar to hers. Present at the meeting were Murray, Allen Steere, Stephen Malawista, chief of the Division of Rheumatology, and Robert Gifford, a Yale rheumatologist who was scheduled to see a woman whose entire family had the disease.

With this fortuitous combination of patient, rheumatologist, and state and federal government representation, the stage was set for researching a cluster of fifty-one cases, including adults and children, who met criteria developed for the first study. The discovery was made quickly that the pattern of symptoms that these patients had, both joint and neurological, were inconsistent with the diagnosis of juvenile rheumatoid arthritis.

A few miles from Lyme, at the Naval Submarine Base New London at Groton, Dr. William Mast, an internist, and Dr. William Burrows, a dermatologist, observed several patients with unusual rashes. When they treated these patients with antibiotics, they noted improvement, validating what they had read about similar rashes in European literature. In 1976, they published an article on four cases in the *Journal of the American Medical Association*. A Yale dermatologist, Dr. Thomas Hansen, had also read the European literature on rashes. When some of Burrows's and Mast's patients had other symptoms in addition to the rash, such as arthritis, they were referred to Yale. The military connection was now added to university, state, and federal involvement in finding answers to the high number of cases of arthritis in Lyme, Connecticut, and the distinctive rashes that were seen by physicians at the Naval Submarine Base New London. At first, no association was made between arthritis, rashes, and ticks.

STUDYING THE NEW DISEASE

Over a period of several years, Allen Steere conducted extensive interviews with Polly Murray in order to better understand the disease. As a rheumatologist, he was more interested in joint problems than in rashes. Not all patients had rashes, and if they did, they had sometimes disappeared by the time patients appeared in doctors' offices. Nor was he convinced of the benefit of antibiotics, as he said in the June 1977 issue of the *Annals of Internal Medicine*. He did not find bacteria in joint fluids and thought the disease might be caused by a virus. However, he searched for bacteria in rashes and continued to study the new illness, becoming known as the pioneer in Lyme disease.

At Yale, Steere began his research by contacting thirty-nine children among the dozens on a list that was given him by Murray. He reached an additional twelve adults also suffering from juvenile rheumatoid arthritis. This was a very large number for the small Connecticut town of Lyme and the surrounding area. (Juvenile rheumatoid arthritis normally affects only one child in a thousand.) About a quarter of the patients remembered a spreading skin rash. Steere learned of a skin rash in northern Europe that was associated with ticks. He also heard about the work of the Swedish dermatologist Arvid Afzelius, who in 1909 described a rash that he associated with ticks. Between 1977 and 2007, Steere published nearly two hundred articles on Lyme disease.

LYME DISEASE IN OTHER PARTS OF THE WORLD

Although the cause of Lyme disease was not identified until several years after Polly Murray brought it to public attention, there was evidence it had been present for at least a hundred years. Documentation in European literature shows that it was by no means a new disease. Because of communication limitations of earlier times, physicians and scientists were less likely to know about discoveries that were made by others, and to make connections between their findings and those of others that would help identify the disease.

In 1883, a German physician, Alfred Buchwald, described a man with diffuse skin atrophy. Twenty-three years later, in 1909, at a meeting of the Swedish Society of Dermatology, the dermatologist Arvid Afzelius presented research on an expanding ringlike lesion he had observed on a woman who had been bitten by a European sheep tick. Aafzelius continued to observe rashes and in 1921 published his work, hypothesizing that the rash came from the bite of a tick.

Benjamin Lipchutz, in Vienna in 1913, described a case of an expanding rash and in 1921 published a report of six more cases in a paper entitled "Erythema Chronicum Migrans." Two years later, he reported a total of sixteen cases. The rash that he first described as erythema chronicum migrans (EMC) became known as erythema migrans, or the EM rash. In 1922 French scientist Charles Garin described a patient with a large EM rash and, concurrently, a neurological disease that would later be related to Lyme disease.

In 1930, the Swedish dermatologist Sven Hellerstrom reported a case of a rash and meningitis and in 1949 presented his findings at a lecture in the United States at the Southern Medical Conference in Cincinnati, Ohio. In 1950, Hellerstrom published an article in the *Southern Medical Journal* expressing his opinion that ticks were involved in this disease. In 1951, he noted the benefit of penicillin for patients who had the rash and who also had meningitis at the same time. After World War II, when penicillin became available, several European researchers were successfully treating the rash with penicillin.

In 1970, for the first time, it was determined with certainty that an EM rash had been acquired in the United States. The man was bitten by a tick while hunting grouse in Wisconsin. The case was reported by Dr. Rudolph Scrimenti, who diagnosed and treated his patient and published his paper in the *Archives of Dermatology.*

In Europe, researchers continued to describe rashes and meningitis. Klaus Weber in Munich reported on a case of EM and meningitis that was cured by treatment with penicillin. In the 1950s, twenty years before the disease was recognized in Connecticut, European scientists were convinced that the EM rash had a bacterial cause. Jonathan Edlow in his book chronicles the discoveries in Lyme disease.[2]

In the United States, this was seen as a new disease which Steere designated "Lyme arthritis." The microorganism that causes it would not be discovered for several years, and its discoverer would be Willy Burgdorfer, PhD. In Switzerland, Burgdorfer was an entomologist doing graduate work with the Swiss Tropical Institute, studying tick-borne infections of interest to military personnel. Ticks were known to be the vector for relapsing fever, and, in 1946 he was given the assignment of infecting ticks with the relapsing fever spirochete and studying the various tick tissues. Over the next three years, he dissected ticks of many types, and during his graduate studies he learned of European dermatologists' belief that the EM rash was caused by a tick-borne disease. He was aware that Hellerstrom had also raised that question, but no one had ever found spirochetes in a sheep tick.

After completing his studies in Switzerland, Dr. Burgdorfer received a fellowship to study at the Rocky Mountain Laboratories in Montana, where he continued to study ticks and spirochetes. He dissected thousands of different types of ticks, explored their physiology, and searched for the many microorganisms that they carry. He became the world-renowned expert on ticks and tick-borne pathogens, including Rocky Mountain spotted fever. Government interest in relapsing fever had waned, and it was no longer a disease of interest. In 1968, however, Boy Scouts on a camping trip in Colorado contracted what was thought to be Colorado tick fever. The Centers for Disease Control contacted Dr. Burgdorfer, who knew that the altitude of the campsite and the season precluded Colorado tick fever and found that the disease was instead relapsing fever. A few years later, in 1973, sixty-two people fell ill after camping in a cabin on the rim of the Grand Canyon, and Burgdorfer identified the cause as relapsing fever.

Meanwhile, a number of scientists searched for the cause of the new disease in Connecticut. Steere spoke with Burgdorfer several times to understand the complexities of ticks and the microorganisms that they carry. In 1981, Burgdorfer examined forty-four ticks and made stained slides. He found that they were free of pathogenic organisms except in the midgut area of two of them. Through the microscope, he saw faintly stained, long, irregularly coiled microorganisms that looked like spirochetes. Their movements were sluggish. He recalled Hellerstrom's article in the *Southern Medical Journal* and Hellerstrom's opinion that ticks were involved in the EM rash. Burgdorfer examined more of the batch of forty-four ticks and found that 60 percent of them contained spirochetes in the midgut. He and his colleagues performed more tests, including allowing infected ticks to feed on rabbits, which, several weeks later, developed skin lesions.

Burgdorfer had identified the spirochete that causes Lyme disease, and his discovery was published in the June 1982 issue of *Science*. In 1983, at the International Symposium of Lyme disease, in New Haven, Connecticut, the Lyme bacterium, Figure 3-1, was named Borrelia burgdorferi in honor of Dr. Burgdorfer.

The Borrelia burgdorferi, known as Bb, is one type of spirochete. Other diseases caused by spirochetes include syphilis and relapsing fever. Although thousands of times larger than a virus, the Borrelia burgdorferi is difficult to see without a powerful microscope. The Lyme Disease Foundation in Connecticut illustrates the small size of the bacteria by saying that fifteen hundred Lyme spirochetes laid end to end would equal one inch. If bacteria were laid side to side, one hundred thousand Lyme bacteria would be required to equal one inch.

The Borrelia Burgdorferi Spirochete

Lyme spirochetes are difficult to culture outside the body in the laboratory. And although in 1982 it was thought that there was only one strain of Bb, there are now known to be at least a hundred strains in

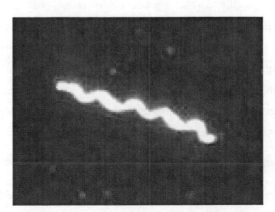

Figure 3-1. Spiral-shaped Lyme bacteria.
Photo provided by Dr. Robert D. Gilmore, CDC.

the United States and three hundred worldwide. A more recently discovered pathogen, identified within the past few years, is the Borrelia lonestari, which causes a "Lyme-like" disease. As with other Lyme Borrelia, it passes from the bloodstream and travels through the body, invading tissues and organs. It penetrates cells and can emerge from them cloaked in a cell's membrane that contains the body's DNA, thus allowing it to avoid detection by the body's immune system.

This characteristic is an important factor in the potential difficulty presented by a case of long-undiagnosed Lyme disease. The bacteria can also exist in a cyst form in which they become dormant and are not responsive to treatment. As are the ticks that carry them, the Borrelia spirochetes are well-adapted for survival.

Spirochetes are long, slender bacteria, spiral-shaped like the coils of a telephone cord, sometimes tightly wound, sometimes not. They are motile with the ability to travel within the body, moving in corkscrew fashion by rotating in place. This is possible because they contain longitudinal fibers that surround the bacterial cells. They move easily in the viscous, gelatinous environments of blood and body tissues, a characteristic that explains the possible wide-ranging symptoms of Lyme disease and the importance of treating it early while it is still localized.

Spirochetes are much longer than they are wide, their narrow width making them visible only under certain microscopes. They divide by transverse fission across their width. The outer membrane of Borrelia burgdorferi is composed of a variety of outer surface proteins, Osp A through Osp F, that are presumed to play a role in virulence. These proteins influence testing methods in diagnosing Lyme because of the immune response that they stimulate, and they are also important in the development of vaccines for preventing the disease.

DEER TICKS

There are more than 850 tick species, and about 100 have been found to transmit diseases. The common dog tick, about the size of a watermelon seed, does not transmit Lyme disease because, although it can be infected with Borrelia burgdorferi, the dog tick cannot maintain the infection as the tick changes stages during its life cycle (see Figure 3-2). The deer tick that transmits Lyme disease is smaller, approximately the size of a poppy seed. Borrelia burgdorferi are located in the tick's midgut, and when the tick inserts its mouth parts into the host to take a blood meal, the bacteria are expelled into the host.

An attached tick cannot be rubbed or scraped off, or pulled out with your fingers. Using Vaseline or a lit match has the effect of causing it to burrow more deeply. Fine-tipped tweezers should be inserted around the head, deep enough so that the entire tick will be removed. The tick should be pulled straight out, at a right angle to the skin. A firm, steady, persistent pressure is required to dislodge it.

The tick that transmits Borrelia burgdorferi is often incorrectly described as an insect. Whereas insects have six legs and three body parts, adult ticks have eight legs and two body parts. Ticks are arachnids, as are spiders, and have four life stages—eggs, larvae (with six legs), nymphs,

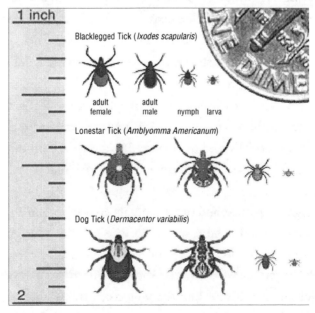

Figure 3-2. Deer tick life stages.
Reprinted with the permission of the American Lyme Disease Foundation.

61

and adults—and require two years to complete them. In the spring eggs molt into larvae. When larvae take a blood meal from a mouse or bird, they molt into nymphs and become able to transmit Lyme disease. When nymphs take a second blood meal from a deer, a dog, or a person, they molt into adults. Females require a third blood meal in the fall, or the following spring, usually feeding on a deer or person, in order to lay eggs. Humans are infected by both nymphs and adult ticks and can be bitten at any time during the year. Although ticks are less active in cold weather, they may bite at any time when the temperature rises much above freezing.

The small black-legged deer ticks that transmit Lyme disease on the East Coast are named *Ixodes scapularis*. The Western black-legged tick, the *Ixodes pacificus*, is found on the Pacific Coast, and in Europe, the tick carrying Lyme disease is the *Ixodes ricinus*. Another deer tick that has been discovered to carry Lyme disease is the Lonestar tick, with a white spot on its back. It is found in Texas and southwestern states and is said to be moving northward. Dr. Fein, from New Jersey, has noted that far more people living in the Northeast have brought in Lonestar ticks than in any other year. One deer can carry a thousand ticks.

Deer ticks have a hard shell that allows them to resist dehydration, and they can live for weeks and months in leafy, shaded areas or inside the house. They depend for survival on sucking the blood of a host: a mouse, or another warm-blooded animal, a deer or a human. Most commonly, adult ticks feed on deer and nymphs feed on mice, and if ticks come in contact with a human, they take a blood meal from a person.

Although deer, mice, and other animals do not become ill from infection with the spirochete, and therefore remain as reservoirs for transmitting the disease, this is not true for dogs and horses, which definitely do get sick with Lyme. If they are bitten by an infected tick, cattle and cats may also exhibit lameness or other symptoms of the disease. Dr. Fein notes that deer have glands behind their knees that secrete a substance that attracts ticks.

THE LYME DISEASE RASH

The Lyme disease rash is diagnostic of Lyme disease and may be the only signal that alerts people and physicians to the fact that the illness is Lyme disease (see Figure 3-3). It is also often the only symptom that physicians will accept for the diagnosis of Lyme. The well-publicized "bull's-eye" rash has a red spot in the center and a clear area around the bite that is surrounded by a pinkish or red ring. Dr. Andy Franks of New York University presented data that less than 50 percent of biopsy positive Lyme rashes are bull's-eyes, also demonstrated in vaccine trials. The rash does not have to be a bull's-eye to be Lyme disease—mine wasn't. It can also be a flat rash that spreads in all directions. It can remain small, or it may expand over a large area, such as across a shoulder, leg, abdomen, or back. It seldom itches or hurts, and the bite is usually not felt because the tick's saliva contains a substance that numbs the skin around the bite.

The common assumption is that a rash always appears after the bite of an infected tick. This is not true. It is observed only half the time. Moreover, the tick also is observed only half the time. You do not have to see either a tick bite or rash, and you may still have Lyme disease.

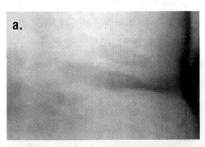
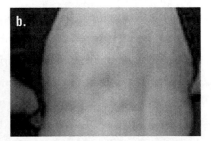
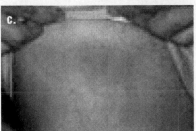

Figure 3-3. Bull's-eye and other Lyme rashes: (a) Multiple Erythema, (b) Single Erythema Migrans with central clearing, (c) Single Erythema Migrans lacking central clearing. *Reprinted with permission of the American Lyme Disease Foundation,* © *2001--05 Dermatlas.*

The rash can appear soon after the bite, many days later, or never. My rash did not appear until the dried-up tick was removed several months later. As the disease progresses, the rash may appear in areas far from the bite site, showing up long after the bite has occurred, as did mine when I discovered several red patches on my chest.

Several years before the bite that made me so sick, I had been bitten by another tick. It could have been attached for no more than twenty-four hours before I saw it on my abdomen. I went immediately to the doctor to have it removed. A tiny area around the bite had already begun to turn pink, but when the tick was removed, the skin returned to normal. I was not offered an antibiotic, and there was no mention of Lyme disease. I didn't know it then, but Lyme bacteria had already been introduced into my body and may be the reason my disease was so severe.

The Lyme rash may be confused with other rashes, and when there is doubt, the rash is sometimes ignored. It may be viewed as a result of a spider bite or an infection other than Lyme, or mistaken for an allergic reaction to an insect bite. Because it may appear as no more than slightly reddened skin, it can be easy to dismiss as local irritation that will go away. It may disappear, either soon or later, and be forgotten. Many people have difficulty remembering whether or not they saw a rash or inflammation. If the skin is red, without a raised, itchy rash, this may not be recognized as a rash, but merely as irritated skin.

In 1982, we finally had information that had been sought since 1975 and which explained the newly identified disease in Lyme, Connecticut. The erythema migrans rash, sometimes called the erythema chronicum migrans rash, was firmly established with the new disease. This was the rash that had been reported by the Swedish dermatologist Arvid Afzelius in 1909 and by Benjamin Lipchutz in Vienna in 1913, who published his paper on erthyma chronic migrans in 1921.

TREATING THE NEW DISEASE

Antibiotics were used for treating the rash before the discovery of the cause of the newly discovered disease. During the early years, interest was on the disease and the study of ticks rather than on treatment. Descriptions of symptoms, and possible chronic illness, were reported in the literature, but the focus did not appear to be on finding the best ways to treat it. This was surprising because it was presented as possibly becoming a long-lasting neurological illness. Treatment, though, became an important part of the history, first surfacing at a Congressional hearing (described in Chapter 7) on the politics of the disease. Lyme became a political illness that involved insurance companies and research grants which seemed to supersede the treatment needs of patients who were ill.

Beginning soon after the Congressional hearing in 1993, physicians who treated patients until they were well, long term if necessary, began to face harassment from insurance companies and medical boards, a situation that continues to this day. As a result of an ongoing aggressive campaign, physician education and the number of knowledgeable physicians available to the public for treating serious Lyme disease is severely limited.

Beginning in the 1980s, Allen Steere at Yale and his colleagues received government grants to continue studying deer ticks, rashes, and the nature of the disease-causing spirochete. Steere, who had trained to become a rheumatologist, became a medical insurance expert for this new disease as well as being a medical researcher. He and his associates and colleagues founded the American Lyme Disease Foundation, which reflected their beliefs. The existence of persisting infection, however, was not accepted by rheumatologists, and it was thought that the disease might resolve on its own. The focus continued to be narrow, mostly on joint symptoms and rash, and did not include the wide variety of other symptoms that can result from infection with Lyme bacteria. The treatment needs of patients did not become foremost, and, in fact, obtaining any treatment at all became the challenge.

Not until 2002, in order to address mounting public pressure, was a treatment study undertaken to address the question of persisting disease. It was a short, three-month study (see Chapter 11) using low-dose antibiotics, conducted by Mark Klempner, who represents the side of the controversy that denies that Lyme disease can become chronic. Excluded in the study were those with a PCR positive for Lyme. Predictably, as a result of its design, the study failed to demonstrate that longer-term antibiotics improved outcome. But despite scientific articles that demonstrate otherwise, it is this study that continues to be referenced by those who do not accept that the disease can persist.

Polly Murray received no treatment for her disease from Allen Steere, other than aspirin, as was true for other Lyme patients. Several years later, still without medical care for her disease, Murray ended her patient relationship with Steere. In 1988, also in Connecticut, Karen and Thomas Forschner, whose six-year old son Jamie died of Lyme disease acquired during Karen's pregnancy, started the Lyme Disease Foundation, with offices in Tolland, Connecticut, where physicians, scientists, and patients come together to study the disease and treatment needs of patients who have Lyme and other tick-borne illnesses.

By 2000, increasing concerns over the spread of the disease, its potential severity, misleading information, and lack of available treatment options for those who are ill led to the formation of two additional Lyme disease organizations. One of them is the Lyme Disease Association, headquartered in New Jersey. The other is the International Lyme and Associated Diseases Society in Bethesda, Maryland, composed of physicians and healthcare professionals. All three organizations play roles in encouraging research, educating the public and assisting those who contract Lyme disease.

I have given the background information on the disease and its nature. The next chapter tells you about diagnosing Lyme. With its arthritic symptoms and neurological complications, it may not be recognized. Indeed, it can be mistaken for one of many conditions. Without a clear-cut clinical picture, treatment can become unavailable for this reason alone.

"IS IT CHRONIC FATIGUE SYNDROME?" "IS IT FIBROMYALGIA?"

DIAGNOSIS OF LYME AND OTHER TICK-BORNE DISEASES

I brought my wife to the doctor and almost had to carry her into the office. She could barely walk and was so weak that she could hardly stand. Her legs were numb and sometimes she had the "shakes," but the doctor said she didn't have Lyme. It took three years and an extensive search to find out she has Lyme disease.

—FEDERAL GOVERNMENT AGENCY ADMINISTRATOR

Stories similar to this one are so common that they can almost be expected at any Lyme disease meeting or conference. If not caught early, the disease can be incredibly difficult for many doctors to identify. In this chapter I will tell you why and will give you a guide to the many possible symptoms and how the disease is diagnosed. There is no one pattern to the illness. Every case has its differences, and the symptoms and course of the disease cannot be predicted. There are, however, common factors. The best you can do is recognize it early so that treatment will more likely be effective and will more likely cure the disease.

As described in Chapter 3 on the history of the new disease, neither diagnosis nor treatment became a priority for those in Connecticut who were studying it. Their many research grants did not focus on the needs of those who were sick, or the antibiotics that might be required to cure them. With the continued denial of serious Lyme by the Infectious Diseases Society of America and the characteristics exhibited by this complex disease, it is not surprising that its diagnosis is often delayed. For many people, the cause of their symptoms will never be known.

My world continued to close around me, even as I tried to keep my life normal and maintain my usual activities. I couldn't explain why I could not keep commitments as I had in the past, and why it was so hard to plan a date and stick to it. For instance, could I drive fifty miles, have lunch with a childhood friend, and tour the historic district? When the morning arrived, I had nausea and called to cancel, but there was no real reason for it that I could identify, and I called back to say that, of course, I could come. By noon the nausea was gone and I was tired and weak. For lunch I ate several salty pickles, used lots of salt, and drank strong coffee to help keep up my strength. On the walking tour I had fleeting burning sensations in my arms and legs.

Then there was my husband's annual summer office party. Could I go? It was hard to believe that I couldn't drive fifteen miles to attend the lobster picnic, but I could not assure myself or my husband that I would be able to. At five o'clock in the afternoon, with considerable hesitation, I climbed into the car and followed the winding road from Wayland to Acton, Massachusetts. I was light-headed and dizzy. At the picnic, to relieve the pain in my knees, I sought a place to sit down, explaining that I had Lyme disease. How did I know? Well, I really didn't. What did the doctor say? Well, I've been to quite a few and they don't seem to know either.

Sometimes I thought a swim in the lake, only two miles from my house, might make me feel better, but my arms were weak and I was very tired. I swam near shore for a short time but couldn't trust my body enough to feel entirely safe and went home. I tried to take walks, but couldn't be sure I could make the return trip back to my house.

Despite my fatigue, I spent many sleepless nights in a living room chair, waiting for first light and dawn. Sometimes I paced the floor. There seemed to be some kind of inflammation in my brain that made me jittery and sometimes left me unable to relax. Where to find answers? There had to be some. I knew this had to be Lyme disease, not some rare disease from some far corner of the earth. But twenty-four doctors had said it wasn't.

I learned later, as reported by the Lyme Disease Foundation and the Lyme Disease Association, and confirmed by my own many conversations with chronic Lyme patients over several years, that the average number of visits required for diagnosis is from twelve to twenty-four. These are representative numbers only for those whose disease is recognized. But many cases never are because physicians have not been given the information they need beyond early symptoms of rash and fatigue, and the Lyme tests (see Chapter 5) are difficult to evaluate.

With my public health experience, I called the Harvard School of Public Health where I was connected to a researcher who said he had been bitten by deer ticks many times without getting the disease. He could not help me. I made nearly a hundred calls around the country searching for answers and inquiring about Lyme disease. I was able to find a few names of doctors who, I was told, treated Lyme, but none would speak to me. Perhaps I didn't ask strongly enough. Office nurses, when asked about Lyme disease, couldn't say much. They said I would have to be seen. There was no indication that I would receive a response any different from those I had already gotten, and there was a three-month wait for appointments. I felt uncertain about my ability to make a trip from my home to Pennsylvania or Connecticut, even lying down in the back of the car. I didn't trust the information and couldn't wait three months. No books explained my dilemma then, and they don't now.

A friend who summered on Nantucket, an island off Cape Cod, became so concerned at my deteriorating health that she investigated Lyme disease on the island. She found a woman named Kim who had personal experience and information on serious Lyme disease, and who was willing to share with me what happened to her.

Despite the high rate of Lyme disease on Nantucket, Kim was caught unaware when she developed chronic fatigue that was so great that her life was nearly shut down. For nine months she sought medical help, first on Nantucket, at the Dartmouth and Johns Hopkins medical centers, where it was suggested she might have lymphoma (cancer of the lymphocytes, which are white blood cells). The recommendation was made that her swollen lymph nodes be biopsied so samples could be examined under a microscope. She had blinding headaches and swollen knees that put her on crutches. Her short-term memory became so undependable that when she traveled to landscape jobs, her husband handed her a piece of paper with the name and address of where she was going. She said she lost a year and a half of her life but was now well and had even run the Boston Marathon. She told me of two others on Nantucket, who, after many months of treatment, had recovered from Lyme disease. She was a beacon of hope. I waited to see her doctor.

I would not recover in a few months as Kim had, and my symptoms weren't exactly like hers, but I was alone no longer. Laid out for me was a course of action that should have been followed months ago. The denial of the diagnosis of Lyme is a major risk for the disease's becoming chronic. This lack of diagnosis occurs even when there seems no credible reason for not recognizing it. And yet it is the common experience that is reported by those with chronic Lyme disease, and they have a stack of medical records to prove it.

Another woman who lives on Martha's Vineyard shared her story and medical record with me.

I saw the doctor in the hospital to whom I was referred by my primary physician. He had my records. He asked me to describe what had been happening to me over the last few years with my health. I brought my friend with me. I said I believed I had Lyme. One of my children was diagnosed with chronic Lyme last year and was put on several months of intravenous antibiotics. I told him I had lived on Cape Cod for several years and had several tick bites and at least one with a rash that spread all over my legs. My symptoms began at that time. I had the flu and my doctor thought I had a virus. My symptoms have waxed and waned ever since. I told him my neuropsychological test was positive for short-term memory loss and loss of train of thought. I described my fatigue and pains that come and go. I told him I thought it could be Lyme.

Our visit went downhill from there. He stopped me and asked if I was there for his opinion or not, and I said I was. He asked why he should believe me that I had a bull's-eye rash when there was no documentation in my records. He said, "You have a bad memory anyway." I was confused because I have short-term memory loss, not long-term.

He did a physical exam and touched several tender points. He said he was sure I did not have Lyme disease, but had fibromyalgia [a chronic condition consisting of unexplained pain]. "They don't know what causes it," he said, "but they suspect an auto accident or viral or bacterial infection." He said my Lyme tests were negative.

Her medical record says,

The patient reports mysterious onset of easy fatigability when she was still able to work. She reports often coming home completely exhausted and needing immediate rest in bed . . . she had diffuse musculoskeletal pains which involved her hands, feet, and muscles of her legs. Her symptoms

71

worsened over subsequent months and years to involve her hips and chest, and she was treated with an exercise program and non-steroidal agents . . . waxing and waning . . . memory problems worsened . . . lapses in work performance . . . she had periods of vertigo which is more described as unsteadiness rather than motion of the room . . . feeling of pressure over the cranium . . . she recalls frequent tick exposure during her youth . . . recalls flulike symptoms with bull's-eye rash.

And her record continues,

"The patient has diffuse musculoskeletal tenderness . . . difficulty in sleeping." The doctor reports on neuropsychological tests done earlier that she had brought with her stating that "the results were partially consistent though certainly not diagnostic of presentation of Lyme disease and that a course of stress management had been suggested at that time. In the past when she presented [came to the office] with the suggestion of Lyme disease, she was given a three-week course of doxycycline with no change in her symptoms following this course of antibiotics."

Dr. Fein notes that Brian Fallon discovered that MRIs did not differentiate Lyme patients from normal controls.

Her report documents normal CAT scans, magnetic resonance imaging (MRI)s, and bone scans done in the past and continues that "absence of positive Lyme serology [blood work] . . . as well as her lack of response to antibiotics in the past are most consistent with a diagnosis of fibromyalgia and less likely to be indicative of a chronic post Lyme disease syndrome." The doctor ends his notes by recommending an antidepressant regimen.

The pain of fibromyalgia can be a symptom of Lyme, but it did not explain her illness. She had been bitten by ticks, had Lyme rashes, pain, fatigue, and experienced short-term memory loss. But no matter what, with every symptom consistent with Lyme, this woman was told that she already had her treatment and did not have Lyme.

The fact that she did not recover in three weeks on the standard antibiotic regimen prevented her from being diagnosed. This happens to people regularly, a result of inadequate treatment and denial of the existence of chronic Lyme disease. Despite the denials, though, Lyme disease, whether early or late, can be diagnosed.

While waiting for my appointment with Dr. Sam Donta, I feared my uncertain symptoms, never knowing what might happen next. It was a challenge to make it through each day, trying to do normal things and finding that I often couldn't. Early in December, the day arrived for my first visit. The neurologist who had admitted me to the Metrowest Hospital had sent my medical records several months earlier. My husband and I arose early for the fifteen-mile journey into Boston, the familiar trip I had made many times as a commuter. This time I prepared as for a safari. I wore green sweat pants, a purple top, and a heavy black-and-white sweater. It was a combination that I knew was odd, but I couldn't seem to do anything about it. I felt very weak and was too sick to decide what to wear. For months I had seldom gotten out of bed. I clutched a bottle of ginger ale and a box of salty crackers "to keep up my strength" and stave off nausea. This, too, felt odd. I wore a heavy coat, boots, and a scarf against the cold.

At the Boston University Medical Center waiting room, I huddled in a chair. I didn't know what to expect and have little recollection of what I said at that first appointment. I answered questions but was too ill to be articulate. I told Dr. Donta about Kim and hoped he would understand and know what to do. He actually listened to what I said. I didn't have to explain much. He anticipated questions that I was too ill to ask. His eyes looked directly into mine and he spoke to me directly, whereas at my many previous appointment the physicians' eyes were always cast downward, looking at my medical records, which showed nothing wrong, while making comments about "her" to my husband. Dr. Donta diagnosed me with Lyme disease.

THE LYME RASH AND DIAGNOSIS

One way that Lyme disease is diagnosed is by the EM rash, as described in Chapter 2. It is the most visible and distinctive symptom, whether or not it is a bull's-eye or spreads from the bite site in an irregular round or oval pattern. If present, it indicates infection with the Lyme spirochete, but you can't count on having the rash because it is observed in only about half of those who get a tick bite. Some have stated that the number is as high as 90 percent, but that high number may be due to the fact that so many cases of Lyme remain undiagnosed.

The Infectious Diseases Society of America, which restricts diagnosis and treatment of Lyme disease, publishes guidelines that are so narrow (limited and specific) that they miss many cases of Lyme disease. For example, because they recommend that a physician-documented rash be required to make the diagnosis, it can be expected that those they diagnose will, by definition, have a rash.

The IDSA statement is "Erythema migrans is the only manifestation of Lyme disease in the United States that is sufficiently distinctive to allow clinical diagnosis in the absence of laboratory confirmation."[1] The guidelines continue, saying that if testing is done, two different tests must be positive to confirm the diagnosis. Both of these tests are unreliable (see Chapter 5).

The Lyme disease organizations, the physicians who treat chronic illness, and their patients, however, know that clinical symptoms and their pattern, beyond the rash and the tests, are diagnostic of the disease. The International Lyme and Associated Diseases Society, the Lyme Disease Association, and the Lyme Disease Foundation estimate that the number of those who observe a rash is no more than 50 to 60 percent.

Furthermore, in addition to not having the rash, only about half of those bitten ever see the tick that bit them. After taking a blood meal, a tick usually drops off, and even with a frequent tick check, it can be missed. It is important to remember that you cannot depend for diagnosis either on seeing the tick that bit you or on getting the rash.

By the time I was diagnosed, my rash had disappeared, but my disease was identified in other ways. My clinical symptoms were strongly indicative of Lyme, and, in addition, everything else had been ruled out. Every test that I had been given was negative.

DIAGNOSING MY DISEASE

When I saw Dr. Donta, I was given the Western blot test for Lyme (see Chapter 5). Two additional non-Lyme disease tests helped to confirm my diagnosis. While all of my standard blood tests were normal, as is expected with Lyme, the antinuclear activity (ANA) reading was high when it should have been zero. The ANA test is used to diagnose lupus, a chronic disease of body tissues. But lupus had been ruled out during my hospital stay. My reading declined over time and after three years of treatment became normal.

In addition to the ANA, I was given the brain single photon emission computerized tomography (SPECT) imaging test that showed reduced blood flow in some areas of my brain. Most Lyme patients do not get the SPECT test, but I found it useful. After three years of treatment, this test also became negative. This change will not occur with lupus or multiple sclerosis, and the fact that both the ANA and SPECT tests became normal after treatment confirmed, in case anyone had any doubt, that I had Lyme disease.

BRAIN-IMAGING TESTS

Brian Fallon in New York is associate professor of clinical psychiatry at Columbia University College of Surgeons, and director of the Lyme disease clinical research program at the New York State Psychiatric

Institute. He has done extensive work on brain imaging in Lyme disease. Among his publications is "A Controlled Study of Cognitive Deficits in Children" in the *Journal of Neurospsychiatry*.[2] He is principal investigator for a four-year study of brain imaging that was funded by the National Institutes of Health and director of the new Lyme Disease & Tick-Borne Diseases Research Center.

Although brain imaging tests will not by themselves confirm the diagnosis of Lyme disease, they may be useful in identifying it, as well as documenting changes that occur during treatment. While electroencephalograms (EEG) show the electrical activity in the brain and may indicate brain irritability, the brain SPECT shows areas of active blood flow and identifies parts of the brain where flood flow is reduced, known as *hypoperfusion*. The SPECT does not show whether reduced blood flow in the brain is due to blood vessel or nerve cell dysfunction, and it may be present in other conditions such as lupus or cocaine abuse, and is therefore not diagnostic for Lyme disease.

The Brain SPECT Test

For this procedure, a radioactive substance is injected into the bloodstream. It emits pulses of energy, making active areas of the brain light up. These are photographed by a camera that sends a series of images to a computer, resulting in three-dimensional photos of the brain. It is an expensive procedure, costing approximately $3,000, and insurance companies may not pay for it. If follow-up scans are done to assess changes, they are done at the same imaging center so that test results can be compared with more reliability.

The Magnetic Resonance Imaging Test

The MRI provides information that cannot be seen on an X-ray, CAT scan, or ultrasound. The MRI uses an electromagnetic field and pulses of radio wave energy to make pictures of internal organs and is useful in diagnosing many illnesses. A magnet changes the magnetic field surrounding the hydrogen atoms in the soft tissues. Unlike the

SPECT, which shows the functioning of the brain, the MRI shows the physical structure of the brain. Dr. Fallon says that in neurological Lyme disease, approximately 15 to 45 percent of patients have white matter intensities as shown in the MRI. The white matter of the brain and spinal cord refers to nerve fibers surrounded by a whitish substance, called the myelin sheath. They are responsible for communication between the gray matter and the rest of the body. The gray matter is found in the cerebral hemispheres which consist of nerve cells and unmyelinated neurons. If the cause is Lyme disease, antibiotic treatment may result in lessening or disappearance of these bright spots on the brain.

The Positron Emission Tomography (PET) Test

PET scans produce three-dimensional images of physiological and biochemical processes that are occurring in the brain. The PET scan is a more expensive procedure than the SPECT, requiring a multidisciplinary staff and high-technology equipment. PET scans are used primarily as a research tool and are not generally available. As in the SPECT, a radioactive substance is introduced into the bloodstream. The resulting images have enhanced resolution and, unlike the SPECT, can provide quantification of metabolic processes and blood flow in different areas of the brain. For children with neurological Lyme symptoms, brain-imaging tests can be useful in assessing a child's ability to attend school.

CHILDREN AND LYME DISEASE

Imaging tests can be useful for other reasons. Children may not be articulate enough to describe their symptoms and how they are feeling. A three-year-old may say no more than, "My knee hurts." Children cannot describe, nor can many adults, exactly what they are experiencing, such as "brain fog," chronic fatigue, difficulty in understanding directions, or remembering what they read. Teachers may see them as listless, inattentive, lazy, having behavior problems. They may do poorly in sports, having little stamina and complaining of pain. It's hard enough for Lyme to be recognized in many adults, but can be especially difficult to detect in children.

Thirteen-year-old Sarah Hale-Rude testified at the Albany, New York, hearing on chronic Lyme disease. Her parents had taken her to many doctors and spent $15,000 out of pocket for expenses that her health maintenance organization (HMO) would not cover.

> My parents took me to many specialists, and all of them found every possible reason to deny that I had Lyme disease. The reason they gave for my being so sick was chronic fatigue syndrome, fibromyalgia, and severe depression. I had already missed a few weeks of school, not having any idea I wouldn't be back for almost a year . . . I was also forced to drop out of the drama club play in which I had a leading part . . . People were accusing me of being a psych case. I had lost my ability to read, my favorite pastime, and every day I felt worse and worse . . . I was falling frequently and hardly able to follow a tutoring session . . . My new family doctor was also quick to suspect a psych problem and reluctant to even consider Lyme disease . . . Of course, my mom had to cancel my place at a sleep-away camp.

More than eight months were required to diagnose her disease. At the time of her testimony a year later, she was nearly recovered and preparing to return to school.[3]

Parents of children with Lyme contact their child's school to explain the absence or erratic attendance of their child. The disease is variable and is not the same for every child. The outcome cannot be assured with any degree of certainty. Parents often must leave jobs to care for the sick children, making some families more vulnerable to loss of medical insurance. School departments must be contacted to determine resources that may be available for disabled children, such as transportation, home tutoring, or home schooling. Services for disabled children vary among school departments and states.

The Lyme Disease Association is a resource on issues that parents of sick children may face, but getting the diagnosis is first and foremost. The problem needs to be known as what it is, and the treatment needs to reflect the cause of the illness. For example, many problems are erroneously ascribed to attention deficit/hyperactivity disorder (AD/HD) or hyperactivity, or the child's lethargy is ascribed to lack of sleep or motivation. Children depend on parents to prevent and recognize their disease. If it is not detected or the correct diagnosis is not determined, the problems of parents and children are very much magnified.

Initial Symptoms of Lyme

The initial Lyme flulike symptoms of fatigue, malaise, neck ache, or headache are often vague and fleeting and may not occur immediately after the tick bite. Although some people have high fevers, most don't. For a few days, I had a mild temperature, for example, when I went to the emergency room of the Metrowest Medical Center early in my disease. Nor was my white cell count elevated as one might expect with infections. Unfortunately, with these two characteristics of Lyme, it is less likely that an antibiotic will be prescribed early, as would more likely occur for other infections. Without the usual indicators, it is not surprising that many cases of Lyme are not treated early or are missed. Physicians who have never knowingly seen a case of chronic Lyme disease may say, "How can she be so sick when all her tests are normal?"

In addition to lack of a fever or elevated white blood cell count, there are other characteristics of the Borrelia burgdorferi spirochete that result in missed diagnosis. Having the disease once does not protect against future infections and often results in the frequent comment, "You've already had Lyme. This can't be Lyme disease." Not only can you get the disease any number of times, but relapses may also occur. Too, it is possible that the disease was not cured the first time, and the return of Lyme symptoms indicates recurrence of the original infection.

MORE SYMPTOMS

There can be wide variability in how the disease presents, making the diagnosis more difficult for those who are unfamiliar with the disease. It is a multisystem illness, meaning that it can affect many parts of the body, depending on where the bacteria travel. As a result, those with Lyme disease typically experience many apparently unrelated symptoms, causing confusion among those who don't know that Lyme disease often presents itself in this way.

In addition to their variability, many Lyme symptoms, with the exception of the erythema migrans rash, can also be present with other disorders. A fast, pounding heart, or irregular heartbeat, muscle weakness, swollen lymph nodes, headaches, dizziness, painful or swollen joints, back pain, gastrointestinal problems, light sensitivity, ringing in the ears, anxiety, depression, fatigue, learning problems in children, sleep problems, could all be symptoms of conditions other than Lyme, and ones that are far more familiar to the public and their doctors.

When informing others that I had Lyme, I was sometimes asked, "How do you know it's Lyme?" If I mentioned sore knees, the question could be, "Are you sure you don't have arthritis?" If I said I had fatigue, the response might be, "You could get more rest." If I said I felt generally ill, the suggestion could be, "You should get a complete checkup."

It was often overwhelming to people when I said that I'd already had, in addition to blood work, a multitude of tests, including MRIs, CAT scans, X-rays, electroencephalograms, and muscle biopsies, and that every test was negative. When asked why my painful knees didn't show up on an X-ray, I explained that the pain and swelling were caused by a spirochetal infection, not by joint or cartilage problems, and infection is not evident on X-ray. Lyme disease does not characteristically cause damage to the joints. When the infection clears, the joints are normal.

LACK OF DIAGNOSIS CAN LEAD TO UNNECESSARY TESTS

Unnecessary tests are costly as well as time-consuming. With the passage of time, and without a diagnosis, insurance companies typically pay for expensive and futile procedures to diagnose conditions that the patient does not have. With the Lyme problem blanketed, insurance companies also typically pay for a wide array of tests, office visits, emergency room visits, and hospitalizations. Nevertheless, some of these tests can be essential because other diseases must be ruled out. It is also possible to have Lyme and another disease as well. When the disease is diagnosed correctly, many of these costs can be curtailed.

Insurance companies have demonstrated that they will pay for these tests rather than reimburse the long-term treatment costs of a persisting disease with its many uncertainties, although other chronic diseases are covered without question. And as would be expected, they prefer to use the Infectious Diseases Society of America restrictive guidelines that limit diagnosis and deny continuing infection. A group of IDSA physicians have long testified as expert witnesses for insurance companies.

Those with Lyme often hear, "You look so healthy." With the exception of the distinctive rash, most symptoms are invisible to others. Inevitably, because the disease is so hidden and so political, frustrated physicians may cast the problem as psychological, and patients are left with stacks of records, many of which state unequivocally, as did mine, that the patient does not have Lyme. Without correct information, people may be put on unnecessary, and even harmful, medications. When steroids are used with undiagnosed disease, they may reduce the body's immune response, and if there is a history of these medications that have been prescribed to reduce inflammation and pain, physicians report that the disease is more difficult to treat.

A Word of Caution

The following pages, in which I offer a cascade of possible symptoms, can evoke disbelief, and the conclusion that the disease is "all in her head." This is reinforced by the variability in different people and in the same person. If there were a single set of symptoms, and if more of them were visible to others, the disease would more likely be accepted for what it is. Especially when laboratory tests come back normal, the possible severity of neurological disease may be attributed to psychosomatic illness or a psychiatric disorder. How many people know that this Lyme disease can cause hallucinations, slurred speech, seizures, periods of paralysis, disordered thinking, schizophrenic behavior, and periods of unconsciousness? It can do all of these things.

The misdiagnosis may be dementia, MS, or Parkinson's. How can you know that it isn't? Common sense tells you to suspect that people who were healthy on Tuesday don't wake up on Thursday with a staggering gait and a diagnosis of Parkinson's. People leading normal lives don't suddenly find themselves unable to read a page, without any known medical reason.

New Symptoms May Appear Later

Not every symptom appears at the beginning of the disease. New ones can appear at any time. For example, during my illness, I occasionally noticed small red spots, called petechiae, that result from bleeding under the skin. They are characteristic of several other illnesses, including leukemia. I had perhaps eight or ten of these spots over a couple of years, all of which disappeared within a few days.

Charles's story is typical. Before becoming ill, he was a lineman in Pennsylvania with the telephone company, working in all kinds of weather. Although he never noticed a tick bite or rash, he discovered that he was losing muscle strength. Many people who were formerly physically strong find that their strength can seem to disappear almost overnight, and that no amount of exercise increases muscle mass or endurance. In fact, for those with Lyme, exercise often results in fatigue from which it is difficult to recover.

Charles became dizzy. If sufferers note feeling light-headed or dizzy, the anti-vertigo medications that are often prescribed seldom provide relief. As time passed, he had difficulty finding the exit from the turnpike to his home and missed it several times. He had memory problems and could not recall the exit number. Sometimes he went east instead of west on the ramp. One day he drove his car into a tree not far from his home.

With a wife and two young children to support, and a mortgage to pay, he was no longer able to work. There seemed no reason for his illness, and none of the doctors he consulted could find one either. He began to sleep eleven hours a day, not wanting to get out of bed to face the vertigo and disorientation. He was given an antidepressant, and that, too, even after many weeks, provided no relief. Most Lyme patients say that antidepressants do not help them.

After six months, with the family in deepening crisis and his wife seeking employment, a fellow lineman recommended a doctor in Pennsylvania. This physician had seen cases of similar disability and suspected that the cause of his problems could be Lyme. He diagnosed him with Lyme disease. Several weeks later, Charles woke one day with a sharp, burning sensation in one toe, the pain so sharp that he could not put weight on that foot. His primary care doctor suspected gout but wasn't sure. His Lyme doctor explained, however, that new symptoms, often very different from the original ones, may arise at any time during the illness, and he recommended that Charles continue his Lyme disease treatment. Within a few days, the pain in his toe disappeared. The sudden appearance of a new symptom is not uncommon and, in fact, is typical, and helps to confirm the diagnosis of Lyme disease.

During Meg's Lyme disease, she developed gastrointestinal symptoms. Sometimes her stomach would accept very little food, and it was difficult to swallow. She often had nausea, a common Lyme symptom, one that I had early in my disease. Although her gastrointestinal special-ist had no answers, digestive symptoms can result from Lyme disease, probably due to neurological disturbance that is caused by infection in the nervous system. Along with gastrointestinal symptoms, she had fleeting muscle pains in her arms and legs. Her eyes became unusually sensitive to light. Her symptoms seemed to make no sense and did not fit the pattern of other diseases. But the uncertain, unexplained pattern can be characteristic of Lyme.

When Meg developed a sore lower jaw and sensitive teeth on one side of her mouth, she called her dentist, asking to be seen right away, fearing an abscess or need for a root canal. By afternoon, the pain had subsided and disappeared. Jaw and tooth pain sometimes result from a Lyme infection. Symptoms that disappear may not be gone forever. They may reappear at any time, lasting a few minutes, or for weeks or months. The unpredictability can make the diagnosis a challenge, es-pecially for those who are unfamiliar with the disease.

Among neurological symptoms may be paralysis of facial muscles, allowing one side of the face to droop as in Bell's palsy. This can result from a stroke, but muscle weakness and loss of sensation, and even paralysis, are also characteristic of Lyme disease. Those with Lyme may say, "I have numbness in my legs," "I can't feel my feet," or "I have no sensation in the fingers of my left hand." The nerves are a favorite lo-cation for the Lyme spirochete. "Burning" sensations are common and may be fleeting. Frequently, for a very long time, my legs felt as though I were walking through hot steam. With the current politics, many neurologists will not be able to diagnose neurological symptoms as caused by Lyme disease. They have not been trained to recognize it if it has progressed beyond early disease. They have been told that Lyme is always cured within a few weeks.

Some people who have these Lyme symptoms, after finding that they do not have one of the chronic neurological diseases with no good prognosis or treatment, have expressed relief in getting the diagnosis, saying "I'm very glad that it's Lyme." However difficult the symptoms, unlike with the chronic neurological diseases, with Lyme there is hope of cure.

MULTIPLE APPARENTLY UNRELATED SYMPTOMS HELP DIAGNOSE THE DISEASE

The common expectation for most diseases is a recognizable pattern, with a course that is generally unique to that illness. The number of possible symptoms in late Lyme disease, and the possible variety, make it almost inevitable that many Lyme patients' problems will be viewed as psychosomatic. All of the characteristics of the disease mentioned above in this chapter help to feed the controversy, and they also help to confirm the diagnosis. Those who believe that too much Lyme disease is being diagnosed can, and do, say, "People get overanxious and think that everything is Lyme disease."

Those on both sides of the controversy, however, accept the fact that Lyme is a multisystem disease with many possible symptoms. But although adherents of the IDSA guidelines accept the existence of varying and persisting symptoms, they resist the idea that the disease can persist beyond a few weeks. Even for heart block, the guidelines recommend no more than a few weeks of treatment. The response continues to be that these symptoms are mostly subjective, perhaps "post-Lyme syndrome" rather than continuing infection. They make the following statement, which has outraged Lyme activists: "Posttreatment symptoms appear to be more related to the aches and pains of daily living than to either Lyme disease or a tick-borne coinfection."[4]

TESTIFYING TO THE LEGISLATURE

Getting diagnosed correctly is a problem that, for many people, has been insurmountable. Some who did finally receive a diagnosis have told their stories at legislative hearings. In 2004, the day following a heavy snowfall that canceled many school classes, I attended a day-long Connecticut legislative hearing on chronic Lyme disease that was organized by the state's Attorney General Richard Blumenthal.

More than three hundred chronic Lyme patients arrived at the legislative building, spilling into the hall and filling an adjoining hearing room. Also present and providing statements were doctors who treat chronic Lyme disease, legislators, state public health officials, and representatives from the Centers for Communicable Disease. All who spoke agreed that Lyme disease is a major public health problem. And as has been true for other state legislative hearings, no physicians representing the IDSA "overdiagnosed" side of the controversy attended or sent written statements to refute the information that was presented.

Among those testifying that day was a teenage boy who said:

> I have had Lyme disease since the summer of 2000 when my mother picked off two ticks from my body, one behind my left knee and the other behind my right ear. I never got a bull's-eye rash. I started having joint pain in the fall of 2000 and was told by my physician I was having growing pains and fatigue due to my intense karate training. I got physically worse and worse as time progressed. I had extreme fatigue that was unrelieved by rest and sleep . . . I had headaches, could not concentrate in school, lost my short-term memory, could not play sports or take karate . . . with my mother's persistence, I had a test for Lyme disease . . . I had a positive ELISA [see Chapter 5]. I received three weeks of doxycycline . . . My symptoms improved and I thought I was well. In October 2002, I had a relapse of symptoms. I felt like I had the flu . . . the doctors at the hospital diagnosed me with joint complications due to the flu . . . my pediatrician told my mom that I could not have Lyme disease because I was already treated for it . . . he diagnosed me with arthritis . . . the infectious [disease] doctor told me my symptoms were all in my head."[5]

In 2001, *New York Times* reporter David Grann interviewed Allen Steere and was invited to sit in on several patient consultations. Steere then led him into a different office and read from a letter dated June 26, 1999, in which a twenty-nine-year-old woman told her story. She was disabled and unable to work, and said she had suffered from Lyme for seven years. She detailed a host of neurological and other symptoms: severe fatigue, muscle pain, low-grade fevers, numbness, palpitations, sinus infections, and more. She described how her life had been turned upside down, including the need to file for bankruptcy.

In the midst of the list, Steere paused and looked up at me. "You've seen some of my patients," he said, "does this sound like Lyme disease?" Steere put down the letter and stared at me for a long moment. "What I suspect is that she doesn't have Lyme disease but some kind of psychiatric illness," he said. "That doesn't mean that I don't care what happens to her." He continued, "We've come to have the idea in America that it's possible to cure anything and that everyone could be well, and it's their right to be well, and they should be angry if the medical profession doesn't make them well."[6]

On November 27, 2001, Five months after the *New York Times* article on Dr. Steere was published, the New York State Assembly Standing Committee on Health held a hearing in Albany on "Chronic Lyme Disease and Long-Term Antibiotic Treatment." Patients and Lyme disease physicians presented testimony and told a very different story from that of Dr. Steere in the *New York Times*. Among those testifying was a former executive for a software company who was stacking firewood at his home when he was bit by a tick, which he discovered several days later. He removed the engorged tick and forgot about the bite. Within a week, he became ill with severe head and neck pain, and a stiff neck. He said,

> I was placed in the isolation ward in a local hospital in Newburgh [New York] as a precaution. The doctors there originally and initially suspected spinal meningitis

or encephalitis of some kind, but testing at that time failed to disclose the source of the illness, and it seemed to resolve itself in a few weeks.

The illness then returned over the following months, causing severely debilitating medical conditions. By 1994, seven years later, I had missed 345 days of work and had spent nearly 100 days in the hospital. Even when not hospitalized, I lived in a constant state of infection. And the doctors were quite puzzled. It was inconceivable that this condition was not improving. By 1994, I was blind in the left eye. I couldn't walk without a cane or a walker. The head pain had become so bad I was unable to function for considerable periods of time. I didn't know family members; I didn't know friends. I had a severely debilitating cognitive dysfunction and required in-home nursing several days a week.

Prior to being sick, I had enjoyed a fulfilling life. I had a very successful career in the software industry. I had been very athletic, spent a lot of time cycling, swimming and running, and here I was disabled.[7]

After seven-and-a-half years, he received a diagnosis of Lyme disease.

Most cases are not that severe, especially when they are diagnosed early, but they can be. Symptoms may be limited to one or two, or there may be many, and they can be mild enough to be largely ignored. The range can be wide and symptoms variable, even in the same patient. Why does someone who develops a swollen knee also develop short-term memory loss and have seizures? What is the connection between a painful shoulder and vertigo? Why does a patient come into the office with a swollen ankle, facial numbness, burning eyes, and fatigue? How can someone who was previously healthy arrive at the doctor's office with leg muscle pain, ringing in the ears, and heart palpitations?

Because Lyme is a multisystem disease with uncertain tests, the diagnosis is primarily a clinical one, with a pattern of complaints that is recognized by physicians who are experienced in treating long-term Lyme. The common theme in diagnosing Lyme disease is that symptoms often appear unrelated and to make no sense. The pattern is that there is no pattern. Nothing in the patient's history explains the problem, and it is this history of apparently unrelated symptoms that assists physicians in making the diagnosis. (See the appendix for a list of possible Lyme symptoms.) Physicians who diagnose and treat chronic Lyme disease rely heavily on the history, the pattern of symptoms, and the total clinical and laboratory picture.

Patients and their physicians need to be aware of factors characteristic of Lyme disease that may derail the correct diagnosis. Before going through a roster of specialists in psychology, neurology, rheumatology, cardiology, and others, people with a number of unexplained and apparently unrelated symptoms might well consider, "Can this be Lyme?"

THE EXPECTED COMMON MISDIAGNOSES

As will be described in Chapter 6, there are far more serious misdiagnoses than chronic fatigue and fibromyalgia, but most commonly those with Lyme disease are told they have chronic fatigue syndrome or fibromyalgia. This occurs so regularly that it can almost be expected. Early symptoms are often "flulike" with fatigue and malaise and include headache and neck ache. Fatigue can be so deep that it often described as "brain fog." If these symptoms occur soon after a tick bite and rash, the diagnosis of Lyme will likely be made. But if the fatigue is long-standing and of unknown cause, the diagnosis may be ascribed to chronic fatigue syndrome (CFS) or fibromyalgia syndrome (FMS) without consideration that these are Lyme disease symptoms.

Both CFS and FMS are conditions for which there are no diagnostic tests and no treatment. No causative agent, such as a virus, has been found for either syndrome, although research is being done. If patients accept CFS or FMS as a diagnosis, without pursuing further investigation, they will not receive antibiotics. Insurers have shown that they prefer the diagnosis of CFS or FMS to accepting evidence that Lyme disease can persist and may require long-term treatment. Both of these conditions are called syndromes and are defined as an association of several clinically recognizable features or characteristics, like "post-Lyme syndrome," that include a combination of typical signs or symptoms.

Diagnostic criteria have been established for both CFS and FMS, but symptoms of CFS often go far beyond the research criteria, to include loss of brain function, depression, and cardiac and respiratory problems. In 2006, the Centers for Disease Control launched a campaign to raise public and medical awareness of this condition.

Chronic Fatigue Syndrome

The story of chronic fatigue syndrome is told by Dorothy Wall in her book, *Encounters with the Invisible*.[8] The description of her disease and her personal experiences with this devastating illness could not be more like Lyme. It is the same story told by countless Lyme disease victims who were initially diagnosed with chronic fatigue syndrome or fibromyalgia and assured that they did not have Lyme disease.

The only treatment for CFS is lifestyle change and medications that address sleep and pain issues, and perhaps the use of antidepressants. Among the many symptoms of chronic fatigue syndrome are memory loss or substantial impairment in memory and concentration, tender neck and armpit lymph nodes, muscle pain, joint pain, sore throat, and headaches. Accepting the research diagnosis for CFS requires at least four of these symptoms that started at the same time, after the fatigue began.

Chronic fatigue is not simple tiredness. Lyme patients know that it appears without warning as a thick blanket of enveloping fog that clouds the mind, prevents thinking, and perhaps even prevents moving out of chair or bed. It is not relieved by sleep, and, when there is sleep, it is nonrestorative. People do not feel rested when they awake.

This syndrome affects more than one million people in the United States. For research purposes, the Centers for Disease Control, where researchers introduced its name in 1988, define it as marked by extreme fatigue that has lasted for at least six months, is not the result of ongoing effort, is not substantially relieved by rest, and causes a substantial reduction in daily activities. It affects people of every age, gender, ethnicity, and socioeconomic group, and it occurs in women at four times the rate of men. Many veterans with the Gulf War syndrome have symptoms that appear almost identical to those of CFS.

Fibromyalgia

Fibromyalgia is the other problematic diagnosis that is frequently given to Lyme patients. When there is no known reason for pain, it is ascribed to this condition. Frequently, it accompanies chronic fatigue syndrome, with many similar symptoms—pain in muscles or joints, tenderness when certain parts of the body are pressed, and lack of energy. For research purposes, fibromyalgia is defined as having widespread pain on both sides of the body, above and below the waist. Tenderness must be present in at least eleven of eighteen points when they are pressed.

Several organizations have been formed to address these two syndromes. Among them are CFIDS (Chronic Fatigue and Immune Dysfunction Syndrome) in Charlotte, North Carolina; the Fibromyalgia Network in Tucson, Arizona; the National Chronic Fatigue Syndrome and Fibromyalgia Association in Kansas City, Missouri; and the National Fibromyalgia Association in Orange, California.

Oftentimes, those who initially receive these diagnoses, after the Lyme infection is recognized and treated, find that their chronic fatigue and fibromyalgia problems resolve. Many who have experience with Lyme disease suggest, with no evidence that proves otherwise, that those who are diagnosed with one, or both, of these syndromes are more likely to have instead undiagnosed Lyme disease. I would not accept either of these conditions as my diagnosis without further evaluation for Lyme disease. Physicians and patients need to be cautious in ascribing symptoms that are characteristic of Lyme to chronic fatigue or fibromyalgia. Misdiagnosis can lead to Lyme disease becoming persistent and chronic.

OTHER TICK-BORNE DISEASES

When Lyme is being diagnosed, other coinfections may also have to be considered. Although Lyme disease is by far the most common tick-borne infection, deer ticks may at the same time carry other diseases in addition to Borrelia burgdorferi, and these may also need to be diagnosed and treated. If any of them are present, recovery from Lyme may be more difficult. For some, the treatment is the same as that for Lyme. Therefore, when Lyme is treated, the coinfection is treated as well.

Coinfections are still relatively unknown to physicians and the public, and reporting requirements, if any, vary among states. Most Lyme patients are not currently being tested for these, and, therefore, the risk and prevalence cannot be determined. Three of the most common ones are babesiosis, ehrlichiosis, and bartonella, all of which may have symptoms that are similar to Lyme.

Babesiosis

Babesiosis is caused by a parasite that can be seen with a microscope. Because it is not caused by bacteria, it cannot be treated with antibiotics that are used for Lyme. It is a malarialike illness caused by a protozoan, a single-celled microscopic organism that has mobility and the ability to invade and destroy red blood cells. Blood transfusions have also been found to transmit this disease.

The first recognized case of babesiosis in Europe was in Yugoslavia in 1957, and the first case in the United States was identified on Nantucket in 1968. It has been reported in Massachusetts, New York, Connecticut, Rhode Island, New Jersey, Minnesota, Wisconsin, Georgia, California, and Washington. Babesiosis is not a nationally reported disease, and many cases are missed because of its similarity to malaria.

In 2004, forty-eight cases of babesiosis were reported in Rhode Island.

Babesiosis symptoms are variable and include headache, fever and chills, night sweats, nausea and vomiting, muscle aches, and anemia. Some people may carry the parasite without symptoms, or they may develop later. Coinfection with Lyme may increase the severity of the disease. Multiple tests may be required for diagnosis because of their unreliability. Babesiosis may be diagnosed by examining blood smears and recognizing the characteristic "ring" form taken by the parasite inside red blood cells. It is treated with drugs that are used for malaria. Treatment can require persistence, taking from three weeks to four months, depending on the degree of infection and duration of the illness, as well as the presence of other coinfections. With Lyme disease also present, babesiosis can be difficult to cure.

Fred had been treated for Lyme disease, with little progress, and recurring Lyme symptoms. He also had severe night sweats and anemia, even requiring blood transfusions. The cause of the anemia was not known until one of his physicians considered the possibility of babesiosis, and the tests were positive. Fred's babesiosis, combined with chronic Lyme, was not easily eradicated.

Ehrlichiosis

Ehrlichiosis, named for the physician Paul Ehrlich, is another tick-borne disease that may be carried by the same tick that carries Lyme disease as well as by the larger dog tick. One type attacks white blood cells called monocytes, and another invades granulocyte white blood cells. It is a bacterial disease that usually develops rapidly and is diagnosed by detecting bacteria directly, or by blood studies, polymerase chain reaction (PCR) testing, or tissue culture. About a third of those bitten by an infected tick have a rash, but it does not develop the circular pattern of the Lyme disease rash. Ehrlichiosis is not yet required to be reported to the Centers for Disease Control, so the number of cases is unknown. It was not discovered until the mid-1980s. Between

1986 and 1997, 1,223 cases were reported in the thirty states that collect information on this disease.

Symptoms of ehrlichiosis are malaise, confusion, severe headaches, muscle and joint aches, chills, cough, nausea, vomiting, and lack of appetite. It is treated with antibiotics that include tetracycline and doxycycline, both of which are used to treat Lyme disease.

Bartonella

Bartonella, sometimes known as "cat scratch disease," is transmitted to cats by fleas and may be present in cat saliva. Bartonella henselae bacteria have also been found to be carried by deer ticks, and it is now known to be one of the possible coinfections that may be present in those with Lyme disease. In endemic areas, where Lyme is especially prevalent, as on Block Island off the coast of Rhode Island, 5 to 10 percent of residents have been found to carry the bacteria. Worldwide, twenty-two thousand cases are identified each year.

Early symptoms are a red, crusted elevated rash at the location of the tick bite, followed by flulike symptoms of fever, muscle and joint aches and pains, nausea, vomiting, and chills. More serious symptoms are encephalitis, seizures, and coma.

None of these often-unrecognized coinfections approaches the amount of Lyme disease that we have, but more research is needed on the role they may play in chronic Lyme disease. Earlier diagnosis of Lyme, with consideration of possible coinfections, would help prevent Lyme disease from becoming chronic.

STATE OFFICIAL CALLS FOR CHANGE

During the same Connecticut legislative hearing, at which the teenage boy described his ordeal, a state official testified about his experience after being bitten by a deer tick. He presented the Lyme dilemma in a strong message with a heartfelt plea for change that is echoed by Lyme patients everywhere.

Five years ago I stood in the building with an i.v. shunt in my arm and it was my fifth year of treatment for Lyme disease. Five years ago I was still suffering with symptoms that inundated every day of my life . . . All I could do was hope and pray that one day I would be well enough to care for my wife and two children. And in part as a result of the [Connecticut] hearing on Lyme disease in 1999 I was able to continue my antibiotic regimen without my insurance company once again denying payment for treatment . . . Now two-and-a-half years later after my last antibiotic infusion, I believe I have finally beaten this disease. I must thank my doctors not for their willingness to treat me but for the courage to stand up for what is right in the face of controversy.

You've heard some very compelling testimonies, and, no doubt, are wondering how our medical community, touted as the best in the world, could allow what has happened to occur. Indeed, the question must be asked: How is it that patients could become so ill, and be misdiagnosed for so long? How is [*sic*] that even after adequate antibiotic treatment, these people can still be infected to the point that active spirochetes are found in their bodies?

Why are there so few physicians who know how to properly diagnose this disease? Why haven't our medical school taught students that Lyme disease can quite often be recalcitrant, difficult?

The science is there, as I believe you will see later on today during the physicians' panel. However, we must depolarize the medical community regarding Lyme disease and accept the truth of the matter.

My hope is that the State of Connecticut will make Lyme disease a true priority. It is, without doubt, a major health threat that has robbed thousands of individuals of their inherent right to live a normal life. I believe the time has come for our state leaders to make serious commitments.

He continued,

> ... [the Connecticut School of Medicine] has a responsibility to impart accurate information to students seeking a degree in medicine. The proof of persistent infection has reached the tipping point in the medical community. And our state's medical teaching institution now has a choice before it. The first choice is to continue with its current methodology of teaching the diagnosis and treatment of Lyme disease. That is using textbooks and other teaching instruments that still, for example, indicate that "the disease, more often than not, presents with a bull's-eye rash." It doesn't. "It will usually be picked up through serological testing." It isn't. "It should be diagnosed using the CDC's reporting criteria." It shouldn't. "It's mainly rheumatological." It isn't. "It requires, at most, a three-week course of antibiotics as the cure." It doesn't, especially when patients have been infected a long time.[9]

With the foregoing information on detecting Lyme disease and patterns of possible symptoms, one would expect that a laboratory test would provide the answers. For a variety of reasons, this is not the case. In Chapter 5, I will explain the available Lyme disease tests, their uses, and their shortcomings.

CHAPTER FIVE

"THERE MUST BE TESTS"

My doctor says my test is negative and I don't need an antibiotic unless I develop symptoms.

—WOMAN WHO HAD JUST SEEN HER DOCTOR AFTER A TICK BITE

T he common assumption is that we have a test for Lyme disease that identifies its presence, as we do for many other infectious diseases. This is not the case and means that the clinical diagnosis, which was discussed in Chapter 4, is of great importance. It requires recognizing that a cluster of unexplained, apparently unrelated symptoms is characteristic of Lyme disease.

If you have had exposure to ticks, simply going for a blood test is not enough. You cannot depend on the results. Dorothy found an attached tick that she could not brush off and went to her doctor, who thought it was a deer tick but wasn't sure. He told her there was no need for a Lyme test and to come back if she developed symptoms. Three months later, she began having fatigue and tingling sensations in her arms. She asked for a Lyme test, and it was negative. Nevertheless, she developed Lyme disease.

The Infectious Diseases Society of America guidelines were written by fewer than a dozen authors who believe the disease is overdiagnosed. These guidelines continue to obstruct progress in Lyme disease, including the testing, thus depriving many of the timely diagnosis that would help to protect their health.

The first IDSA guidelines were published in 2000. The second guidelines in 2006 remained largely unchanged from those of 1993. They were produced with Gary Wormser as lead author, with many of the same group of signers as in 2000: Raymond Dattwyler, Eugene Shapiro, Allen Steere, Mark Klempner, and Robert Nadelman, all of whom have published extensively their views that Lyme disease is over-diagnosed and overtreated.

Despite the epidemic, and mounting evidence of persisting disease, the 2006 guidelines are even more restrictive than previous ones. When they were published, the response from the Lyme community was immediate. The Lyme disease associations and support groups across the country, including Tennessee, Indiana, California, and other states, initiated a massive effort to challenge the guidelines.

POLITICS AND THE DIAGNOSIS OF LYME

Richard Blumenthal, Connecticut's attorney general, initiated an un-precedented investigation into the development process of the IDSA guidelines, claiming that scientific evidence that did not sup-port the authors' conclusions was ignored. Among the controversial recommendations, in addition to requiring a physician-documented rash, is the requirement of two positive tests. No test diagnoses Lyme with an acceptable degree of reliability. It is the unreliability that, along with variable symptoms, enables the disease to remain undiag-nosed. Treatment decisions cannot depend on observing a rash or re-ceiving a positive test result.

Whereas for many diseases, blood tests, X-rays, CAT scans, MRIs and ultrasound procedures result in a diagnosis that is generally ac-cepted as definitive, as we know, for Lyme disease these standard lab-oratory tests are all generally negative. Furthermore, as described in Chapter 3, neither the tick nor the rash is observed more than half the time, helping to ensure that many cases will not be recognized.

But, however unreliable, Lyme tests play a part in diagnosing the disease. They do not show the bacteria. Instead, they are indirect, meaning that they assess the body's immune response, which is the production of disease-fighting antibodies. The antibodies that are produced help to confirm the presence of a Lyme infection. Direct detection of Borrelia burgdorferi is difficult or impossible because the bacteria cannot be easily cultured except under specific laboratory conditions, and are unlikely to be found in blood, urine, and body tissues. They cannot be found predictably in spinal taps. Spirochetes have been identified, however, in localized Lyme rashes before they have disseminated into other parts of the body, and they have been seen in autopsy.

Despite this information, "post Lyme syndrome" continues to be hypothesized as a possible autoimmune disorder, or psychosomatic disorder, something that requires research money. A *Newsday* article in 2007 says, " Raymond Dattwyler [one of the group of physicians who denies chronic Lyme] said the government has thrown a lot of research money at studying persistent infection associated with Lyme disease, but the bacteria just aren't there after the acute infection is treated."

The article then says [of the Klempner study that denied chronic infection and that is used by the insurance industry], "Klempner said he and his colleagues took samples of spinal fluid, blood and urine, searching for evidence of active infection. 'Over 750 lab exams,' Klempner said, 'And not a single person at any point in the study had evidence of the bacteria.'" The article continues, "'They are suffering something, but it isn't persistent infection,' Dattwyler says of the unexplained neurological and physical problems."[1]

With this view of a disease that is not always cured in a few weeks, those who don't get well promptly can face challenges in acceptance of their diagnosis. They then may be exposed to the accompanying risk of not receiving comprehensive treatment for their disease. Accepting a negative test result when other indicators are present means taking a chance.

DISCOVERING A TICK

Ellen's doctor removed an attached tick from her back, noting a small red area around the bite. He swabbed it with alcohol and decided there was no need for a test. She had no symptoms at the time but has vague feelings of uncertainty about her health. She wonders if she should have a test now. Many would say yes, because, if it is positive, she would more likely have access to an antibiotic. And whatever the result, there would be information that could be useful in making a future diagnosis. In any case, it would have been safer for Ellen to take a preventive antibiotic, especially because the Lyme rash indicates that she has Lyme disease.

A number of differing scenarios may occur. Jim asked for an antibiotic when a tick was removed from his leg. Unlike Ellen, he was given a test, and the result was negative. Because his doctor didn't want to give treatment without a positive test, his request was denied. He wonders now whether delayed treatment affected the severity of his disease.

TESTING THE TICK

Although the spirochetes cannot generally be found in body fluids or tissues, they can be detected in ticks. If a tick is not infected, you do not have Lyme disease. State health departments or university laboratories sometimes provide a service where ticks can be tested, but this option is limited. Private laboratories, for a fee, may offer tests for Lyme and other tick-borne diseases. You put the tick in a sealed plastic bag—do not put it in alcohol or it cannot be tested—and mail it to the laboratory. The result comes back to you or your doctor in about a week. I have used this service for a member of my family who was bitten by a tick. The tick should also be tested for babesia, bartonella, Rocky Mountain spotted fever, ehrlichia, and mycoplasma.

STILL NO DIAGNOSIS

Surprisingly, even with a confirmed positive test performed on the tick itself, the Lyme diagnosis may not be made. Barbara was bitten by a tick that her primary care doctor sent to a state laboratory. It tested positive for Lyme disease, so her doctor put her on an antibiotic and referred her to an infectious disease specialist in case she needed further treatment.

The second doctor gave Barbara a Lyme test that was negative and decided that, although the tick had the infection, it had not yet transmitted the disease. This conclusion is not backed up by facts. A negative test does not mean that she was not infected. And, while it is possible that the attached tick had not yet injected spirochetes into her blood, it's unlikely that she was safe from the disease, and it wasn't worth taking the chance. The doctor, though, said she didn't have Lyme and took her off the antibiotic. Today, she has chronic fatigue syndrome.

THE IMMUNE SYSTEM

Antibodies are proteins found in blood or other body fluids and identify and neutralize foreign substances such as bacteria and viruses. They are Y-shaped and composed of units called chains. The general structure of all is similar, but there are variants allowing antibodies to detect a wide variety of infectious agents.

Because of former infections, the blood may contain antibodies that are not the result of Lyme bacteria but are present due to other previous infectious agents, thereby giving a false signal that a test is positive. As well, if antibodies have not yet formed after introduction of the bacteria into the body, the result may be a false negative. If the disease has become chronic, the spirochetes may no longer be in the bloodstream. They may have traveled to the brain and other body tissues where they more easily evade the immune system and antibiotics.

The immune system is a collection of mechanisms within the body that allows it to detect a wide variety of agents, including tumor cells. It enables the body to distinguish them from its own healthy cells. Lyme spirochetes may be in cyst form, inside cells, or cloaked in the DNA of host cells as they emerge from their intracellular location. In this case, no antibodies will be produced, and test results will show a false negative. Those without antibodies in their blood may actually have more infection.

TWO TESTS FOR LYME

The two scientific tests that are used to identify Lyme disease are the enzyme-linked immunoabsorbent assay (ELISA) test and the Western blot. Other tests exist in laboratories but are not available to the public. Polymerase chain reaction tests that amplify and identify DNA are difficult and costly and are not reimbursable by insurance companies. Knowing what these tests are, and how they are performed, helps you to understand their uses and their limitations. Other tests, such as the C6 peptide assay, may be performed.

The ELISA Test

The ELISA test, the most commonly given, is the one that is the least costly and the least reliable. It measures the immune response to the Lyme bacteria. In the laboratory the spirochetes are placed in contact with the patient's blood serum. If the blood contains antibodies to Lyme disease, the antibodies will bind to the Borrelia burgdorferi proteins. The bound antibodies are detected when a second solution is added and a color change takes place. The ELISA test picks up no more than a third, perhaps half, of the cases of Lyme disease.

The Western Blot Test

The Western blot is a better test than the ELISA, diagnosing about two-thirds of the cases of Lyme disease. Dr. Sam Donta finds that 75 percent of patients showing negative results for Lyme disease with the ELISA will test positive with the Western blot. The Western blot uses Lyme bacteria cells that have been disrupted with electrical current and a detergent. The electrical current separates the Borrelia burgdorferi in a gel, and the proteins are blotted on paper. The proteins separate according to molecular weights measured in kilodaltons (kd), with heavier proteins traveling at a different rate from lighter fragments.

The fragments are then exposed to the patient's blood serum with an added enzyme solution, and if a specific protein is present, a band will form on the immunoblot (the Western blot). The laboratory report will contain two parts, the IgM bands and the IgG bands, two types of immunoglobulins in the blood that are produced by the immune system to fight disease.

There is general lack of understanding of antibodies and Lyme tests. Donta says, "The IgM is the first antibody system to respond to a foreign substance, usually within the first 5–10 days. IgG antibodies begin responding 10 days or so later, and can last for long periods of time, i.e., years, especially if boosted by repeat exposures. The IgM antibody response should disappear with resolution of the infection. If, however, the infection persists, the IgM antibody may also persist, which is what I think is the case in chronic Lyme disease. Using the IgM and IgG antibody systems for diagnosing the presence or absence of the disease is not very accurate; in the case of Lyme disease, there are no other currently available tests, so some people have relied on the IgM and IgG tests."[2]

The types and numbers of bands help diagnose the infection. There is disagreement over how many bands and which bands constitute a positive test. Some bands are given higher diagnostic criteria than others. The 31 and 34 kd bands are known to be strongly indicative of Lyme, and yet many commercial labs do not report them. They were removed from criteria by the CDC. Donta finds that the 23 kd protein and the 41 kd protein appear to be diagnostic of Lyme, and, although the 23 kd band is not unique to Borrelia burgdorferi, it does appear to correlate with Lyme, and, if present, diagnoses the disease. This band, however, is not seen in every case of Lyme.

He adds, "Most symptomatic patients have positive immunoglobulin IgM Western Blots consistent with active, chronic disease. With the resolution of symptoms the IgM reactions may disappear or attenuate. Dr. Fein noted that IgM antibodies may persist despite remission. IgG reactions may continue to be present with resolution of symptoms, but they typically attenuate or disappear with successful therapy."[3]

Most people are never given the Western blot. And, for those who do have it done, many with chronic disease never have even one positive band. The problem is not only the test itself, but the way the test is performed, and how results are interpreted. Sometimes faint bands may not be counted. Laboratories may use different strains of the spirochetes and perform the test in different ways. The same sample sent to different laboratories may yield different results. Physicians have said, "I find that I get more negative results from some laboratories than others. Sometimes, in the same laboratory, it seems to depend on which technician evaluates the sample."

Donta provides the most complete explanation of the testing procedure that I have seen, helping to clarify the puzzling limitations and inconsistencies in laboratory results for the Western blot.

> The Western Blot is a qualitative test, i.e., no real quantification, whereas the presence or absence of reactions results from one lab to the next depends on several factors:
>
> a. How much of the serum [from the blood specimen] was actually transferred to the test tube containing the other reagents and buffers; it's usually a very small amount (50 microliters) and although the pipets used for the transfer are accurate, the technician doing the test might transfer more or less than the 50 microliters.
>
> b. There is only one dilution of the serum usually used (usually 1:100) so, again, dependent on the amount of sample transferred and the accuracy of the dilution, results might vary greatly.
>
> c. The strips that are used for the Western Blot contain the proteins of the Lyme bacteria against which the serum (containing the antibodies) is being tested; depending on how those strips are prepared, and their

ability to be stored over time at various temperatures are probably the major reasons for variation from lab to lab.

d. The type/strain of borrelia might influence test results; there continues to be debate as to whether geographic differences in borrelia strains might influence the reactivity. Some labs use multiple strains to the same Western blot; others use different strains.

e. The reader of the tests might choose to read a band as being negative if not intense enough a reaction; others might grade the response as faint, mild, moderate, or intense, and grade these responses. I've advocated calling the response present or absent, as there is no obvious correlation between intensity and numbers of responses with disease intensity.

Because the Western blot is a qualitative test that describes and evaluates the procedure with no real quantification that can define the disease, it becomes possible for politics to play a role in diagnosing Lyme disease. With its strongly opposing views, including whether or not it can become chronic, the struggle cannot be anything other than intense, with Lyme victims and the public as the stakeholders in what happens in diagnosing and treating the disease.

In order for a small group of powerful physicians with lucrative grants to control medical care for a widely prevalent disease, it is necessary to protect their position and avoid lawsuits. To accomplish this, disagreement or dissent is eliminated. The tactics can be brutal, including denigration of victims and investigation of physicians who treat chronic Lyme disease. The attacks continue, as they have ever since testimony on chronic illness was first presented at the congressional hearing in 1993. Incredible as it may seem, in 2006, three more Lyme disease physicians faced loss of medical license for overtreating Lyme disease.

THE LABORATORIES AND THE POLITICS

With this knowledge, it can be expected that laboratories are not immune to the controversy over the diagnosis of Lyme. Current tests are open to interpretation, and, as a result, laboratories that diagnose the disease can find themselves in the midst of the politics. Those that diagnose "too much Lyme" may result in scrutiny by their state's licensing authority. IgeneX Laboratory in Palo Alto, California, is a pioneer company in diagnosing Lyme and other tick-borne diseases. When it came to attention in 2003, the purported reason was that the number of Lyme cases diagnosed was "too high," although there is no number that can be identified as "too high." The assumption appeared to be that test results from the laboratory could not be accurate.

On June 8, 2005, the *New York Times* reported on a case in which a patient of Gary Wormser, lead author of the most recent IDSA guidelines, was given a negative result but received a positive result from IgeneX Laboratory. To people who know about the differences in performing the procedures and the interpretation of results, this is not uncommon and would not come to any attention if politics were not in play. Differences might be accepted, but those with the view that the disease is overdiagnosed are quick to note laboratory results that run counter to their own assessment of the disease.

An earlier incident involving the laboratory was announced at the Lyme Disease Foundation Conference in April 2000. Nick Harris, IgeneX president, reported that it had refused a sample sent by Mark Klempner, also a member of the IDSA guidelines subcommittee, because the sample had been handled improperly. But what particular incident may have precipitated investigation of the laboratory's procedures is not known.

As a result of the investigation, the patient advocate Lyme organizations initiated a nationwide letter-writing campaign in support of IgeneX. Its reputation was restored, and IgeneX, licensed in New

York as well as in California, remains a major diagnostic and education resource for tick-borne diseases.

The search for a better test continues, but sometimes promising leads are not pursued. In 1998, Ronald Schell, PhD, of the University of Wisconsin Medical School, developed what appeared to be a promising borreliacidal assay test that might differentiate current infection from past exposure, and which was more accurate than current ELISA tests. He sought to have it approved by the Food and Drug Administration (FDA). But Raymond Dattwyler, among the signers of the IDSA guidelines, and adviser to the FDA and the Centers for Disease Control, noted that his own patented ELISA-based test had already received FDA approval, and, as reported by the Lyme Disease Foundation of Connecticut, the CDC decided not to pursue Dr. Schell's test. Physicians on the IDSA side of the controversy have claimed that the ELISA test done in their laboratories is more accurate than others, but many patients have found this not to be true.

The U.S. Centers for Disease Control and Diagnosing Lyme

Another factor limits acknowledgment of Lyme disease. The Centers for Disease Control developed a standard for the specific purpose of providing uniformity in reporting the number of Lyme disease cases. In many ways it was, and is, somewhat arbitrary. It was necessary to define requirements that all could use when reporting cases. As the CDC, however, states unequivocally, the standard was never designed to provide the basis for the diagnosis. Surveillance criteria should not be used for this purpose. And yet they continue to be used, mistakenly, to diagnose Lyme disease. Significantly, they disregard the importance of the 31 and 34 bands in diagnosis.

The Infectious Diseases Society of America uses this standard to diagnose Lyme disease, which is a Lyme rash, followed by a positive ELISA test, followed by a positive Western blot. The CDC surveillance standard is what the IDSA has defined as necessary to acknowledge and treat the disease, and these guidelines are posted on the CDC Web site. If they, rather than the guidelines of the International Lyme and Associated Diseases Society, are used, the combined effect, though not the intent, of limiting diagnosis is increased numbers of people with late-diagnosed, persistent disease. Many with serious, crippling Lyme cannot come close to meeting this standard, and if it is used, it is estimated to miss at least half the cases of the disease. The surveillance criteria and IDSA guidelines allow insurance companies to deny claims for Lyme disease that would otherwise be impossible.

Despite recent efforts by the Lyme disease organizations, the ILADS guidelines, which better protect patients, are not posted on the CDC Web site. The ILADS guidelines for medical care for Lyme disease say, "Since there is currently no definitive test for Lyme disease, laboratory results should not be used to exclude an individual from treatment. Lyme disease is a clinical diagnosis and tests should be used to support the diagnosis rather than supersede the physician's judgment."

In addition, surveillance requirements have not been updated to reflect what we now know about Lyme disease. Because Lyme was originally thought to be limited to the Connecticut region, the CDC requires exposure to occur in an area endemic for Lyme, not acknowledging that the disease now occurs throughout the United States. And because earlier symptoms that were noted in Lyme, Connecticut, were arthritic in nature, it requires, for example, one or more swollen joints, not taking into account that many have no arthritic symptoms, but have disabling neurocognitive symptoms. Although this may soon change, CDC criteria do not yet include the neurological symptoms that Brian Fallon and other physicians have described, including the most common symptoms of chronic fatigue and fibromyalgia, that are almost universal in Lyme disease.

Also required is the presence of a physician-documented rash of at least five centimeters, meaning that the appearance of a rash must be noted in a person's medical record. Laboratory confirmation of the diagnosis with a two-tiered assay is a requirement as well. This means that the ELISA test must be given first, and be positive before the more accurate Western blot can be given. On the Western blot, there must be five positive bands. Since we know the unreliability of the tests and uncertainties of observing the rash, logic tells us that many cases will be missed.

Not all laboratories report every band of the Western blot test. The ILADS provides a warning statement, saying, "The Western Blot should be performed by a laboratory that reports *all* bands related to the Borrelia burgdorferi. Laboratories that use the FDA-approved [Food and Drug Administration] kits, for example, the Mardx Marblot, are restricted from reporting all of the bands, as they must abide by the rules of the manufacturer. These rules are set up in accordance with the CDC's surveillance criteria.

By limiting the number of bands, there is increased risk of false-negative results. The commercial kits may be useful for surveillance purposes, but they offer too little information to be useful in patient management. Two of the excluded bands are 31 kd and 34 kd, which are known to be strongly indicative of Lyme disease.

Neither doctor nor patient may be sure of the best course of action, or how much risk is involved by doing nothing. If a test is ordered, the conclusion that is drawn may be erroneous. If the test result is positive, because of the test's known unreliability, it may be ignored as a false positive, with the remark, "You can't trust Lyme tests." On the other hand, a negative test result may lead to denial of treatment by physicians who don't understand the tests, even if the person has symptoms. Furthermore, if a false negative test result is accepted as correct, and the disease progresses to require more extensive treatment, the person may be denied adequate insurance reimbursement.

What to Do After a Tick Bite

The often-asked question is "I had a tick bite and a rash. Should I have a Lyme test or should I wait for other symptoms?" Because a deer tick bite and Lyme rash are diagnostic of Lyme disease, whatever the test shows, the result does not change the diagnosis. If you have the rash, you have a Lyme infection.

Another question is, "The test is unreliable, so should I take a preventive antibiotic just in case?" The critical question, though, is whether or not a test should be given when an attached tick is discovered, and, importantly, whether the test result should determine the treatment decision. Physicians who have formerly been reluctant to give a preventive antibiotic to their patients, or perhaps have prescribed only a single dose of antibiotic, have been questioned about what they would do for their families. Their answers have been, "If it were my child, I would give the test, and an antibiotic, at least a week, and probably more." Increasingly, this is being done, but it is often necessary for those who want preventive treatment to make this request to their doctors. It's a question of acceptable risk.

Sometimes reported is "My doctor says the tick was not attached long enough to give me Lyme disease." There is no way to know whether a tick has been attached long enough to transmit it, or whether the tick is infected, unless you have it tested, and that requires at least a week. The number of hours required for transmission of the disease, whether four, eight, twelve, twenty-four, forty-eight, or seventy-two, cannot be determined with any certainty. Most people don't know how long the tick was attached, nor can they assess whether or not it is engorged with blood. Ticks begin to feed immediately, and the longer they feed, the greater the risk. Carrying Lyme disease and coinfections that include babesiosis and ehrlichiosis, along with a host of other pathogens, they have been described as "cesspools of infection."

The ILADS guidelines for Lyme say, "Antibiotic therapy may need to be initiated upon suspicion of the diagnosis, even without definite proof." In its summary it says, " Since there is currently no definitive test for Lyme disease, laboratory results should not be used to exclude an individual from treatment. Lyme disease is a clinical diagnosis and tests should be used to support rather than supersede the physician's judgment. The early use of antibiotics can prevent persistent, recurrent, and refractory Lyme disease."

We don't know many of the answers, but we do know that one test may not tell the story. During my search for a diagnosis, I had two negative ELISA tests and one negative Western blot. After several months of treatment, my Western blot became equivocal, showing faint bands that some technicians might have ignored. After a year-and-a-half of treatment, my Western blot came back strongly positive with at least seven bands, including those that are most indicative of Lyme disease. A possible reason may be that aggressive antibiotic treatment reached the sequestered bacteria, bringing them out of hiding, and making them more available to antibiotics and my immune system. Eventually the number of my Western blot bands decreased, and I stopped having the test done. Dr. Fein's 1996 study, presented at the Lyme Disease Foundation Conference, found that of patients diagnosed with chronic neurologic Lyme, 30 percent were seronegative at the first visit. Within nine months of treatment, 90 percent became seropositive.

I didn't know why my persistent disease was denied by every physician I saw, despite the evidence, and the reasons for its apparent trivialization. If I hadn't had any symptoms, or had become well in a few weeks, I would not have known how serious Lyme disease could become, or how often it is misdiagnosed. The following chapter tells you what can happen to those who depend on tests and whose Lyme disease is not detected.

CHAPTER SIX

"IF IT ISN'T LYME, WHAT IS IT?"

THE CONSEQUENCES OF NOT DIAGNOSING LYME DISEASE, MULTIPLE SCLEROSIS, ALZHEIMER'S DISEASE, LUPUS, AND MORE

My husband was diagnosed with early Alzheimer's three years ago, and his memory problems got worse. He lost his job, and we anticipate the need for residential care. My older son did well in early grades, but now can't keep up in school or do sports. He has asthma that he never had before. He had several seizures and was also diagnosed with epilepsy. My other son was diagnosed with hyperactivity and attention deficit disorder. I had Lyme disease with a rash and was cured, but I have so much fatigue that I can't be up more than a couple of hours a day, and am told I have chronic fatigue syndrome. Our whole family is sick.

—ATTENDEE AT A LYME DISEASE CONFERENCE

This family's story is not unusual as we know from the information on Lyme disease symptoms in Chapter 3. Over several years, ticks were brushed off or pulled out, in their lush yard and when they vacationed at the New Jersey shore, or removed from the dog. They enjoyed an active outdoor life until they became ill, and all of them sick in different ways. Only after seeing a news report did they suspect Lyme. With the help of a specialist, who treats late-diagnosed disease, they all are recovering, including the husband who was misdiagnosed with Alzheimer's.

CRITICAL FACTORS THAT MAY RESULT IN MISDIAGNOSIS

This family's experience could hardly be otherwise given the unreliable and misunderstood tests that prevent recognizing the disease, and those who deny that it can last more than a few weeks. When cases are pronounced, "It can't be Lyme," or "It can't still be Lyme," they will not be counted, and medical treatment will not be available If these cases persist or recur, they more often than not are given other diagnoses and names, and that is exactly what is happening. "There are a lot of people out there who think they have Lyme disease but don't," says Raymond Dattwyler, one of the signers of the Infectious Diseases Society of America guidelines. "We are not serving these people well . . . they are suffering from something, but it isn't persistent infection."[1]

This view was reinforced by the American Neurology Association, which issued new nervous system disease guidelines in May 2007 demonstrating support for the Infectious Diseases Society of America and the overdiagnosed, overtreated side of the controversy. It said that it "found no compelling evidence of a beneficial effect from the prolonged use of antibiotics in post-Lyme syndrome." A *Medscape* article quotes from the ANA's statement: "It's clear that patients have symptoms that are very disruptive to their lives, and it's clear it's not infection, but it's not at all clear what it really is, and we need to figure out a way to answer that question."[2]

TOO MANY REPORTED LYME CASES

At its June 2007 meeting in Atlantic City, the Council of State and Territorial Epidemiologists (CSTE) infectious disease committee introduced a proposal to revise the Lyme disease national surveillance definition. The purpose is to limit the number of reported cases. The stated reason for new recommendations is the need to reduce the Lyme surveillance burden on the states. The number of Lyme cases has nearly doubled since 1991. If the recommendation to redefine the disease more narrowly is adopted, its appearance on the Web site of the Centers for Disease Control will minimize and marginalize the epidemic further. Even more cases will be missed and CDC criteria already don't catch at least half of them.

The Council of State and Territorial Epidemiologists proposes that the CDC surveillance criteria (see Chapters 3 and 4) require cases to be defined either as *confirmed* or *probable*. For a case to be confirmed, one of the following would be required: (a) a Lyme disease rash with known exposure to Lyme disease, (b) a case of EM that has laboratory evidence of infection where there is no known exposure to Lyme disease, or (c) a case with at least one late manifestation such as cognitive impairment that has laboratory evidence of infection.

"Known exposure" is defined as less than, or equal to, thirty days before onset of EM in wooded, brushy, or grassy areas, in a county in which Lyme disease is endemic. "Endemic" has been defined as a place in which "at least two confirmed cases have been previously acquired, or in which established populations of a known tick vector are infected with Borrelia burgdorferi."

A definition that includes the requirement of "known exposure" raises several questions. With a growing epidemic, who knows how many ticks are infected in counties nationwide unless resources are available, with a program that is in place, to count and test them? There is also no way to know how many cases have been previously acquired in a county. In many areas, reporting can be almost nonexistent. State reporting is far from adequate, especially where the disease is less known. Heard often is "We don't have Lyme disease here" when this is no longer true. Definitions and redefinitions of what makes the disease reportable could not happen if we had a trustworthy test.

The characteristic rash alone diagnoses Lyme according to the International Lyme and Tick-borne Diseases Society, and this definition is generally accepted if the rash is identified as a Lyme rash. The surveillance criteria do not need to include the requirement of exposure in an "endemic area." To be counted as a case of Lyme, the revision says it must include exposure in an endemic area that is defined with arbitrary numbers, and without the needed facts to make the determination.

As we know, many people with Lyme—and that number is estimated to be at least half—will never have a rash. To meet the requirements for diagnosis, a lesion must be a physician-documented round rash that expands over a period of days or weeks and is required to reach at least five centimeters in size. The Lyme disease rash has specific characteristics but size varies greatly from small, faint, and barely there to one that covers, for example, the entire shoulder.

The proposal says, "For most patients, the expanding EM lesion is accompanied by other acute symptoms, particularly fatigue, fever, headache, mildly stiff neck, arthralgia [pain in joints], and myalgia [pain in muscles]. These symptoms are typically intermittent." Many Lyme patients will tell you that these symptoms came later after they had a rash that was ignored. Symptoms may or may not be intermittent.

The council says, "Laboratory confirmation is recommended for those with no known exposure." This means, however, confirmation with a test that is known to be unreliable. In all confirmed cases a positive test is required, although the fact is that many with Lyme disease will never have a positive test. The only exception is when the rash that meets the definition occurs in an area defined as endemic.

According to the council's proposed revision, planned to be in place by 2008, there is a third possibility for reporting Lyme, a case that has at least one late manifestation, or rash, that has laboratory evidence of infection. A rash, as we have said, is diagnostic of Lyme. Late manifestations, as written, are severely restrictive, but, for the first time in surveillance criteria, neurological symptoms, such as meningitis, palsy, and encephalitis, are acknowledged and included. "Headache, fatigue, paresthesia [numbness, tingling]" and "pins and needles" or mildly stiff neck alone, however, are not criteria for neurological involvement, which means infection of the central nervous system [brain and spinal cord] or peripheral nerves. Again we meet the laboratory testing problem. The recommendation requires either a positive laboratory culture for Borrelia burgdorferi, or two-tier testing that includes first a positive ELISA, followed by a positive Western blot (see Chapter 5).

And these are only the neurological symptom exclusions, meaning symptoms that do not meet the criteria for case definition for reporting the disease. There are others for arthritic symptoms. Among the arthritic exclusions are "recurrent, brief attacks (weeks or months) of objective joint swelling in one or a few joints, sometimes followed by chronic arthritis in one or a few joints." Also excluded are "chronic, progressive arthritis, not preceded by brief attacks, [occurring on both sides of the body], and chronic symmetrical polyarthritis [occurring in many joints]." These are major exclusions. They are common arthritic symptoms of Lyme and therefore should be included.

There are also major cardiac exclusions that are common Lyme symptoms and should be included. Accepted are "acute onset of high-grade second- or third-degree atrioventricular [chambers of the heart] conduction defects that resolve in days to weeks and are sometimes associated with myocarditis. Palpitations, bradycardia [heart rate under sixty beats per minute], bundle branch block [interference with the heart's electrical conduction as shown on the electrocardiogram], or myocarditis [inflammation of the heart muscle] alone are not criteria for cardiovascular involvement." At least 10 percent of Lyme patients have cardiac symptoms.

The suggested change by the Council of State and Territorial Epidemiologists of no longer accepting the rash alone as diagnostic of Lyme, except in endemic areas, strikes at the core of the science. We cannot depend on current tests. We know that antibody production may not occur in Lyme, especially early in the disease when the body may not have yet mounted an immune response. Symptoms often do not occur for an uncertain length of time. Those who are bitten by a tick are better served by taking an antibiotic immediately, and not waiting for symptoms to develop. This requires a physician prescription, and it should be possible to get one, despite the prevailing controversy and misinformation. Waiting for test results to come back from the laboratory makes little sense. The clinical requirements of certain Lyme symptoms, but not others that are equally disease-related, are confusing to patients and their physicians.

THREE PROPOSED CATEGORIES

The case definition establishes three categories for reporting purposes. They are confirmed, probable, and suspected. In addition to the *confirmed* cases, the *probable* category case definition is designated as "any other case of physician-diagnosed Lyme disease that has laboratory evidence of infection," and, again, there is the testing problem. (Both sides of the controversy agree that we don't have a gold-standard test.) Suspected cases would be defined as those with laboratory evidence of a positive test but no clinical infection, meaning symptoms such as seizures or palsy.

Should you fall into the suspected category by having a positive test, you would, of course, want to take a preventive antibiotic. This does not mean that symptoms have appeared, but, in any case, most people would not wait for them before taking a preventive antibiotic. Though Lyme is a multisystem disease that includes many possible symptoms throughout the body, nowhere do we see this definition of it included in the proposed revision. And although guidelines for probable and suspected cases do not require that they test positively on the Western blot test, people are not being treated just because they do not have a positive test.

With the complexities of these three categories, physicians can be expected to have a difficult time in evaluating and reporting Lyme disease to their state health departments. The requirements are so detailed and specific that cases may be even less likely to appear in Lyme statistics than they are now.

The newly proposed CDC criteria of these categories for reporting Lyme disease that will be submitted to the CDC are designed for surveillance only, exactly as are the current ones, saying that "the surveillance case definition was developed for national reporting of Lyme disease; it is not intended to be used for clinical diagnosis." But as occurs now, this tends to become the standard for diagnosis for those who are following, whether knowingly or not, the IDSA guidelines. Although Lyme disease is primarily a clinical diagnosis, there is no category for clinical diagnosis in the reporting system.

To report a case, a definition that addresses the need for uniformity must be developed, and for some diseases this is difficult. It should be designed so that it does not exclude common characteristics of the disease or require tests that will miss at least a third of the cases. Knowing the reporting story of restrictive and complex case definitions helps those with possible Lyme, and their physicians, to avoid costly delay and possible misdiagnosis.

The Council of State and Territorial Epidemiologists plans to send case data to the CDC for all *confirmed* and *probable, but not suspected,* cases. And only fully identified information will be released by the CDC to the general public. "Other releases require signed data-sharing agreements using a format preapproved by the state/territorial agency."

On June 27, 2007, Lyme patients held a rally at the convention center in Atlantic City to protest the revisions. They objected to the continued use of two-tiered testing that prevents diagnosis of Lyme by depending on two unreliable tests, and the exclusion of common Lyme symptoms in the case definitions, saying the changes will make it harder for Lyme patients to get diagnosed. They were told by a CSTE spokesperson that their concerns were unfounded. Because the CDC usually accepts recommendations of the Council of State and Territorial Epidemiologists, it is especially important that patients and physicians become aware of the problem of using CDC criteria for diagnosing Lyme disease.

RESULTING MISDIAGNOSES

With each hurdle that is erected—from more unreliable tests to continued attempts at definitions with too much specificity—more people with Lyme are put at risk of being told mistakenly they have multiple sclerosis or Alzheimer's disease. These misdiagnoses can, of course, have far more serious consequences for patients and their families than those of chronic fatigue syndrome, fibromyalgia, "post-Lyme syndrome," a possible autoimmune disorder "that we don't yet understand," psychological problems, or being told that their disease has already been cured, "Just because you have symptoms doesn't mean you still have active disease."

Lyme bacteria can invade the brain, often resulting in brain swelling, as with meningitis or encephalitis, that may cause "head pressure," "brain fog," or short-term memory loss. Older patients are sometimes assumed to have had a stroke. Depression, hallucinations, thoughts of suicide, behavior and personality changes may occur with Lyme, and patients are sometimes misdiagnosed with bipolar disorder. Reports come from parents saying a child was thought to have autism because of symptoms that were actually caused by Lyme. And when the child was treated, the symptoms improved or disappeared.

Since the IDSA holds that Lyme doesn't persist beyond a few weeks, late Lyme is less likely than early Lyme to be diagnosed correctly. If people are sick with Lyme for a longer time than a few weeks, they can expect the diagnosis to change. And for those whose disease was never recognized in the first place, even with the tick and the rash, it may be more threatening than "post-Lyme syndrome." For example, joint pain may be ascribed to incurable arthritis.

A New Hampshire woman says, "I was told at a Boston hospital that my arthritis was progressive and I should expect to be in a wheelchair within a couple of years. I couldn't believe it. I had never had joint pain before. As far as I know, my blood tests and X-rays were normal. I'm only thirty. I live near a conservation area which has deer. I called my veterinarian, and everyone else that I could think of to find help. I found a Lyme doctor and was cured in four months, but I have nightmares thinking about what could have happened to me."

Robert Bransfield, a New Jersey psychiatrist and board member of the International Lyme and Associated Diseases Society, lectures and writes about neurological Lyme disease. Amiram Katz, MD, a neurologist in Connecticut and assistant professor of neurology at Yale University, lectures on Lyme and the brain. Virginia Sherr, a Pennsylvania psychiatrist and ILADS board member, has published articles on the physical and psychiatric effects of Lyme disease. Brian Fallon, an associate professor of psychiatry at Columbia University and director of the Lyme & Tick-Borne Diseases Research Center, publishes and lectures on the various aspects of neurological Lyme disease and has done treatment studies on the benefits of antibiotics in treating chronic Lyme. All are well aware of the misdiagnoses. In light of the evidence that physicians find, the American Neurology Association's decision to follow the IDSA guidelines is seen as a step backward.

Patients have faith in their doctors and trust the diagnoses they are given, but it's not about faith or trust. It's about both patients and physicians having information they need to prevent this potentially serious and misdiagnosed illness. People who have been misdiagnosed with multiple sclerosis and other diseases have told their stories to local news outlets, sometimes to national media as well, but the public and their physicians remain largely unaware of what can happen with this disease.

Lyme, an illness that can be treated, shares common symptoms with other neurological diseases that are progressive, and even fatal, and diagnoses of these diseases, discussed below, can be problematical as well.

Lou Gehrig's Disease: Amyotrophic Lateral Sclerosis (ALS)

Fred, who is now cured of Lyme disease, says,

> How could they have made this terrible mistake? How
> could they have jumped to a diagnosis that was hopeless
> without even considering what else it could be? I asked
> them about Lyme. Why do they say there is no such thing
> as chronic Lyme disease? I sold my business, changed my
> will, moved out of my house, and prepared for my death
> because I had a progressive fatal disease. My muscle weak-
> ness got worse. My speech was affected, and I was told I
> would be dead within two years. But my condition re-
> mained stable, and I didn't die, and only then did I find a
> doctor who diagnosed Lyme disease.

Amyotrophic lateral sclerosis is only one of the possible diseases
for which Lyme may be mistaken. Although not the most common
misdiagnosis, its effect on lives is comparable to the misdiagnosis of
Alzheimer's. More commonly known as Lou Gehrig's disease, for the
baseball player who died from it in 1941, amyotrophic lateral sclerosis is of Greek origin, meaning "no muscle nourishment." About five
thousand cases of ALS are diagnosed each year.

In ALS, motor neurons in the brain and spinal cord degenerate and
die, ceasing to send messages to muscles, which then atrophy. The onset of the disease may be slow and at first not noticeable. For example,
weakness in a leg may cause stumbling or awkwardness. Arm or hand
weakness may prevent performing simple tasks such as unlocking a
door. As months go by, more muscles atrophy. Standing and walking become no longer possible, and arm and hand movements are lost. Stiffness and twitching may occur. Although cognitive functioning remains,

speaking and swallowing are difficult, and breathing eventually requires mechanical assistance. Depending on the location of the disease, these late symptoms may occur earlier, but wherever the disease appears muscle weakness and atrophy spread; the brain becomes unable to send messages to muscles. A motor disease, ALS does not ordinarily impair vision, hearing, taste, and smell, or the ability to feel touch. Death often occurs from pneumonia and inability to breathe due to atrophy of respiratory muscles.

The cause is unknown, and in 95 percent of cases there is no family history. It occurs worldwide, affecting all races and ethnic groups, most often in those from 40 to 60 years of age. Associated factors are exposure to neurotoxins, a possible virus, or immune or enzyme disorders.

What matters to Lyme patients is that there is no definitive test for the diagnosis of ALS, and symptoms are similar to those of other neurological disorders, including Lyme. Its diagnosis, as is Lyme's, is primarily based on clinical signs and symptoms that are observed by a physician. Laboratory tests are performed to rule out other diseases.

An electromyography (EMG), a test that detects electrical activity in muscles, is given. A nerve conduction velocity test may be done, also a breathing test. A magnetic resonance imaging test may be normal in ALS but is done to identify other possible conditions. Lyme can mimic or present with features of ALS, as can other neurological diseases, and the Lyme diagnosis can be missed.

Multiple Sclerosis (MS)

Marie entered the hotel lobby walking awkwardly on crutches after a two-hour drive on the interstate. She came to the morning session of the Lyme disease conference in Philadelphia, where she said, "I have a hard time traveling because I have urinary incontinence and have to plan for that. I also need to find a chair; my balance isn't good." She added that for five years she thought that she had multiple sclerosis but was now on antibiotics for Lyme and seeing improvement. Because her symptoms were those of multiple sclerosis, the many doctors she saw never even considered Lyme. "I was left untreated for all those years. I don't remember a tick bite, but I live in Pennsylvania where we have one of the highest rates of Lyme disease."

Patients and physicians report that multiple sclerosis, a central nervous system disease that affects nerve cells in the brain and spinal cord, is the most common misdiagnosis among the neurological diseases that are later found to be chronic Lyme. Surrounding some of the neurons in the nervous tissue is the myelin sheath, which is a fatty layer that helps transmit electrical information. In MS, it is destroyed in a process that is known as demyelinization. An inflammatory process results in attacks on the myelin sheath by the body's immune system, and multiple scars (scleroses) are produced. In the early stages of the disease, it may repair itself, although with a thinner layer of myelin. The most common theory is that MS is an autoimmune disease, but the cause is unknown, and a viral or bacterial cause is being considered.

Magnetic resonance imaging of the brain and spine is used to evaluate suspected MS lesions, caused by demyelinization, will appear as bright spots. These white, bright spots may also occur in Lyme, but in Lyme disease, with successful treatment, they may disappear. Two further tests may help diagnose multiple sclerosis. A lumbar puncture can be done to collect a spinal fluid sample, which may show the presence of oligclonal bands, immunoglobulins (antibodies) that indicate chronic inflammation. (These may also be found in some other conditions.) A third test, the evoked potential test, measures the speed of impulses along neurons. This response to stimuli may reveal demyelinization. Slow brain response to stimuli may reveal demyelinization.

MS is diagnosed mostly by symptoms and is difficult to recognize in its early stages. Attacks are often brief and mild. It has been defined as requiring two anatomically separate demyelinating (loss of myelin sheath surrounding nerves) events occurring at least thirty days apart. A definitive diagnosis cannot be made until these have taken place. The most common early sign is a change in sensation in arms or legs, muscle weakness, and vision problems. There can be unsteadiness in walking and difficulty with balance, depression, severe fatigue, visual impairment, overheating, and pain. Some people have already developed several problems when they are diagnosed.

As is common with Lyme, symptoms wax and wane and may disappear, only to recur. They come as attacks in which symptoms come and go, or the disease slowly progresses. The degree of disability varies among individuals. Those whose initial symptoms include difficulty in standing and walking have a poorer prognosis, but some cases progress slowly, with many remissions. People with MS may continue to lead normal, or nearly normal lives, and it is reported that one out of three will still be able to work for fifteen or twenty years.

It is most common in northern geographic regions far from the equator, occurring mostly in Caucasians. It typically appears between the ages of 20 and 40, and in northern Europe, continental North America, and Australia about one out of a thousand individuals suffers from it. It occurs more often in women than in men. Lyme, too, occurs more often in women, twice as often, and may be more difficult to treat. In Lyme patients with an MS-like presentation, the female predominance may be due to the presence of estrogen that makes the environment more favorable to the spirochete.

MS was first recognized by Jean-Martin Charcot as a clinical disease in 1868, although others had described the illness. The three signs, known as Charcot's triad, are speech problems, coordination difficulty, and tremor. Describing it, he mentioned "enfeeblement of memory" and "conceptions that formed slowly." All of these symptoms are shared with Lyme disease, thereby opening the possibility of misdiagnosis.

PARKINSON'S DISEASE

Jean-Martin Charcot named this disease for the British physician James Parkinson, who first described it in his 1817 "Essay on the Shaking Palsy." The changes in the brain that cause it were identified in the 1950s, and in 1967 L-dopa treatment first came into clinical practice.

In Parkinson's disease, the myelin sheath is not destroyed as in multiple sclerosis, nor do motor neurons degenerate and die as in ALS. It results from a loss of dopamine-secreting cells in one part of the brain, the substantia nigra, the "black substance." Dopamine is a neurochemical transmitter, and with its loss, there is decreased stimulation of the motor cortex of the brain, and therefore movement becomes impaired. Abnormal proteins that are associated with damaged nerve cells also appear. Parkinson's is one of the movement disorders that disrupts motor skills and speech.

Symptoms can be many, and include tremor, rigidity, increased muscle tone, slowness or absence of movement, and postural instability. There can be a shuffling gait, problems with speech, swallowing disturbances, fatigue, difficulty rising from a seated position, impaired coordination, dizziness, and slowed reaction time. There are also non-motor neurological symptoms such as short-term memory loss, and cognitive disturbances that may progress to dementia. Symptoms include insomnia, digestive disturbance, and pain in muscles and joints. For most cases, there is no specific cause. For some there can be associated risk factors that include a genetic factor (meaning that it runs in the family) and head trauma (past episodes of head trauma are reported more frequently than by others in the population); a recent study has shown that those who have experienced head injury are four times more likely to develop the disease. There is also drug-induced Parkinson's disease and Parkinson's that results from exposure to toxins. Although it was known long before the Industrial Revolution, it was not until the early nineteenth century that its later symptoms were noted.

The toxins most strongly suspected are certain pesticides, and some metals such as manganese and iron. In a longitudinal cancer prevention study, individuals exposed to pesticides had a 70 percent higher incidence of Parkinson's than those who were not exposed. A substance similar to the opioid MPTP (1-methyl, 2,3,6-tetrahydropyridine) that contaminated heroin was responsible for a string of Parkinson's disease cases in California in 1982, and was subsequently used to induce Parkinson's in animal studies. PCBs, paraquat (herbicide) rotenone (insecticide) and organochlorine pesticides, including dieldrin and lindane, have been linked to it and studies show that those who consume rural well water, which is more likely to be contaminated with agricultural chemicals, have a higher rate of Parkinson's disease.

No blood or laboratory tests have been proven to help diagnose it. CAT scans and MRIs also do not diagnose it. The Parkinson's Disease Rating Scale is the primary clinical tool used for diagnosis. Its progress is variable among individuals, and as with other neuromuscular diseases, its course is unpredictable. It is a chronic, progressive neurological disease, but treatments are available to alleviate symptoms. By itself, it does not cause death, and the disease may progress over a period of many years, with varying courses among individuals. Unlike with ALS, the life span is nearly normal. Death may occur from pneumonia, choking, or as the result of a fall.

Parkinson's shares symptoms with Lyme, and, therefore, Lyme can be misdiagnosed as Parkinson's disease.

LUPUS

Lupus Erythematosus are Latin words meaning "wolf" and "red rash." Named during the Middle Ages, lupus, like Lyme, is one of several chronic diseases that are described as being the "great imitator." Because it is a multisystem disease, it can be misdiagnosed as arthritis, multiple sclerosis, and other illnesses. The first useful treatment, quinine, was discovered in 1894. During the mid-twentieth century, steroids began to be used. Several useful medications are now available which include immune suppressants, antimalarial drugs, corticosteroids, and non-steroidal anti-inflammatory drugs (NSAID). Treatment is aimed toward preventing "flares" (temporary increase in symptoms) of the disease and includes lifestyle changes such as avoiding sunlight.

Symptoms vary widely, depending on where the disease attacks, which is most often the skin, joints, heart, lungs, liver, kidneys, and nervous system. Lupus is an autoimmune disease in which the immune system attacks tissues and cells, resulting in inflammation and damage. The body's normal physiological functioning is disrupted. There can be fatigue, pain, abdominal discomfort, and fever. Lupus's flares are prevented by minimal use of steroids. Their long-term use is associated with obesity, diabetes, elevated blood pressure, cataracts, and osteoporosis. Fortunately, 90 percent of lupus patients can expect to have a good quality of life and now survive more than ten years.

Criteria for diagnosis have been established, including the number of symptoms that must be present for purposes of classification. The American College of Rheumatology has established eleven, although there are more. For a person to be eligible for clinical trials only four symptoms are required, which must occur during a given period of observation. These include a positive antinuclear antibody blood test, a red skin rash (malar rash) across the nose and on the cheeks, blood cell disorders, oral ulcers, sensitivity to ultraviolet light, pericarditis (inflammation of the membrane surrounding the heart), pleurisy (inflammation of the membrane around the lungs), non-erosive arthritis in two or more peripheral joints, kidney disorder, seizures or psychosis, red scaly patches on the skin, and a variety of abnormal blood chemistries.

Those whose relatives have lupus are at a slightly higher risk of contracting the disease. It appears to be more prevalent among women of African, Asian, Hispanic, and Native American origin, although causative factors are unknown. Young women are nine times more likely than men to be diagnosed, although in men and children lupus may be more severe. It is estimated that between 270,000 and 1.5 million people in the United States have the disease.

According to Dr. Fein, Lyme disease is the first bacterial infection known to induce systemic lupus erythematos in both humans and animals. In BALB mice, if you infect them with Bb, they test positive for lupus and not Lyme.

ALZHEIMER'S DISEASE

Alzheimer's, sometimes described as senile dementia, is probably the most well known now among the neurological diseases. Amyloid plaques, protein fragments, which are normally produced by the body, aggregate between brain cells to form a hard, insoluble substance. Other chemicals, which are broken down in healthy brains, are also involved in its formation. Amyloid plaques and neurofibrillary tangles—twisted nerve fibers that form inside the brain cells of Alzheimer's patients— are diagnostic of the disease, yet can be identified only on autopsy.

Although a definitive diagnosis of Alzheimer's can be done only after death, as the disease progresses, psychological tests can provide evidence. Diagnosis is made primarily on the basis of a person's history, clinical observation, memory tests, and intellectual functioning over a series of weeks or months. Blood tests are used to rule out other diseases, and neuroimaging tests may play a supportive role in indicating dementias. Not all dementias are due to Alzheimer's. Tests focus on memory, attention, abstract thinking, the ability to name objects, and other cognitive skills. These differentiate Alzheimer's from temporary impairment, perhaps due to depression, or from psychosis.

For most of the twentieth century Alzheimer's disease was diagnosed in individuals between the ages of 45 to 55. Later onset disease was considered to be a normal part of aging, perhaps due to "hardening of the arteries." Today we understand the primary risk factor for the disease is advancing age.

When it was first studied in 1901, Dr. Alois Alzheimer, a German psychiatrist, interviewed a woman brought to his office by her husband. Initially he recorded her illness as "amnesic writing disorder." Alzheimer later worked in the laboratory of Emil Kraepelin in Munich, Germany, who believed that neuropathology could be linked to clinical psychiatric function. When the woman he had interviewed died in 1906, Alzheimer worked with two Italian physicians to examine her brain anatomy and neuropathology. He then presented to the Assembly of Southwest German Psychiatrists his description of the amyloid plaques and neurofibrillary tangles in the brain that are associated with the degeneration of nerve cells.

In 2004, Alzheimer's was the seventh leading cause of death in the

United States, with 65,820 deaths. More than five million Americans are estimated to have the disease; most have no clear family history and the rare examples that have a familial component usually occur at an early age. Genetic investigations are under way to identify genes that relate to chemical changes in the brain. Alzheimer's has been linked to the first, fourteenth, and twenty-first chromosomes. Today, among people who are age 65, 2 to 3 percent of the population show signs of Alzheimer's. At age 85, 25 to 50 percent of Americans have symptoms of the disease. Risk-reducing factors include intellectual stimulation, physical exercise, and good diet, but these may not alter its progression after symptoms have become evident. Nor do current treatment drugs slow the progression, except in early disease for some people. Most of the answers that we need on prevention and treatment of Alzheimer's are not yet available. Lyme disease, with its shared symptoms, can be misdiagnosed as Alzheimer's.

COMPARING LYME DISEASE DIAGNOSIS WITH OTHER NEUROLOGICAL DISEASES

It is accepted that multiple sclerosis and other neurological diseases do not have a definitive test and that standard blood tests do not diagnose them. Symptoms are variable and unpredictable. They flare and then become quiet. The course is not the same in every individual. Patients are usually diagnosed clinically, with the focus on the history and pattern of symptoms, exactly as Lyme is diagnosed.

For other diseases, patients do not have to go to twelve to twenty-four doctors to get their illness recognized, as they do for Lyme when it has progressed beyond the early stage. Symptoms for other diseases are accepted as being variable and involving many parts of the body. Patients with other illnesses are not told on their first visit that their symptoms are "all in their heads." Their doctors don't say, "There's no evidence you have lupus." They are not left for months and years with pain, fatigue, difficulty in walking, with "fibromyalgia" or "chronic fatigue syndrome" in their medical records. These patients don't have to prove their illness, or the fact that they are sick. Their doctors don't challenge them with the words, "What makes you think you have multiple sclerosis?"

Because of the political controversy, the diagnoses of other neurological diseases appear to occur more easily than the diagnosis of Lyme, and sometimes these diagnoses should instead be of Lyme. Though Lyme has many of the same symptoms as these other neurological multisystem diseases, somehow Lyme is often excluded at the outset. Patients often typically hear, "Your test is negative." "That's not a Lyme symptom." "That doesn't look like a Lyme rash to me." "You've had this for six months? It can't be Lyme." "I've already given you one antibiotic refill." "Yes, I've heard there's a controversy, but I don't know what it's about. I'm sure you don't have Lyme."

Paul Mead, medical epidemiologist for the Centers for Disease Control, says, "Unfortunately, Lyme disease has become an answer for a lot of people. You can't blame them for wanting to have an answer and particularly one where there is hope of treatment and therapy and a cure, but I fear sometimes people fall into a trap of accepting Lyme disease as this broad diagnosis that could explain any symptom."[3] Dr. Mead attended the January 29, 2004, legislative hearing on chronic Lyme disease in Hartford, Connecticut, where patients and their doctors testified on what happened when Lyme was not diagnosed and the disease became chronic. He spoke on Lyme but did not respond to the patient testimony.

Those who claim the disease is overdiagnosed speak of "evidence," saying, "There is no evidence." Cases that are presented are categorized as "anecdotal." There is talk of "isolated incidents." Never mind that much medical practice is of necessity based on a limited number of patients, such as reports that are published in a medical journal on a series of patients, or on uncontrolled trials. Sometimes, in regard to a drug, new or not, patients are offered a medication, perhaps from the physician's desk drawer, with the suggestion, "Try it and see if it helps."

We have evidence of undiagnosed and chronic Lyme disease, and research that supports it. Although there are those who deny that the disease can become inactive, and then become active again, the characteristics of the spirochete are well known. They replicate slowly. They are not always active and can change into inactive cysts that can be reactivated. They can remain inside cells where they are protected from the immune system and antibiotics. An analogy can be made with tuberculosis, a disease that if incompletely treated comes back.

"I had three misdiagnoses before I was diagnosed with Lyme. Why is it that doctors don't learn from their mistakes? Why don't they have to face legal consequences? Why is the medical profession not accountable for diagnosing late Lyme as something that it isn't? It seems that by eliminating the diagnosis that, in effect, they deny the disease. They should consider Lyme first, not last. For me, they never considered it at all." This came from a man attending a national Lyme conference whose graduate studies had to end because of his disease. His frustration is that of so many who feel let down by the medical profession in regard to this potentially disabling illness. Unlike other neurological diseases, treatment, perhaps long-term, is required for Lyme.

NEUROLOGICAL LYME DISEASE COSTS MONEY

Lyme disease requires antibiotics, and many of them do not penetrate the blood-brain barrier effectively. The blood-brain barrier, discovered by the bacteriologist Paul Ehrlich at the end of the nineteenth century, is composed of endothelial cells that line the capillaries. In the brain these cells are more tightly packed, protecting the brain from a large number of chemicals in the blood. The result is that many therapeutic medications cannot be transported easily to the brain. In biological terms, the barrier protects the brain from bacterial infection. However, many viruses, and Lyme spirochetes, can penetrate it.

To increase their effectiveness, intravenous antibiotics have long been utilized for the treatment of Lyme disease, especially for neurological symptoms. When delivered directly into the blood, they bypass the digestive system where some of the medication is lost. Some antibiotics may be delivered both intravenously and orally. Daily infusions of the medications, however, are costly for insurance companies. IDSA physicians and insurance companies have, therefore, often limited the treatment duration to no longer than four to six weeks for Lyme. This short time may be effective for early-diagnosed disease but has been found insufficient for treating cases requiring several months or more. Daily infusions for other conditions, including long-term conditions, are expected to be covered by insurance. Chemotherapy, as an example, used for cancer patients, will not be questioned, but for Lyme disease the situation can be different.

THE IDSA POLICY OPPOSING LONG-TERM TREATMENT

Those with possible Lyme disease face obstacles from every possible direction. Attempts are made to define it narrowly, limit its treatment, and even eliminate doctors who treat it the way it may need to be treated. The resulting misdiagnoses interfere with early treatment that can prevent long-term, costly illness.

After Lyme's identification, Allen Steere was involved in all aspects of the new disease. He became the acknowledged expert. From the outset, however, he and others who are associated with writing the Infectious Diseases Society of America guidelines have consulted for insurance companies and served as expert witnesses in court for companies who deny medical insurance coverage to Lyme disease patients. These physicians also testify for state medical boards against Lyme disease physicians who treat chronic disease.

One of these physicians, Eugene Shapiro, has been a witness against Charles Ray Jones, the foremost pediatrician with the most experience nationwide in treating children with long-term, serious disease. In one of his news comments Shapiro said of Lyme patients, "They'd rather have Lyme disease than multiple sclerosis. They'd rather have Lyme disease than depression which carries a stigma. They'd rather have Lyme disease than something nobody can figure out."[4]

WHAT TO DO

If you've had a tick bite, or have symptoms of and could have been exposed to Lyme disease, consider it first, not last. If, during the past few weeks, or even longer, you've been outdoors in long grass, beach grass, leaf piles, or shrubbery, or walked along narrow woodland paths, or had exposure to pets that have been in these areas, you cannot exclude the disease. You're far more likely to have Lyme than to have developed arthritis, multiple sclerosis, or Alzheimer's.

If the rash or cluster of symptoms indicate Lyme, most people will not want to take the chance of waiting. Other neurological, cardiac, and rheumatologic diseases may be considered and ruled out. Their initial assessment may be no more accurate than the assessment with Lyme, and accurate diagnosis may take time. Certainly someone with a Lyme rash may elect to take antibiotics rather than visit several specialists over a period of weeks or months in case it might be something else. As always, the decision depends on the degree of risk the person is willing to accept.

WHY MANY PATIENTS ARE NOT RECEIVING THE DIAGNOSIS THAT THEY NEED

We know that restrictive guidelines and unreliable tests obstruct the diagnosis of Lyme disease. The politics of Lyme disease and the polarization between the two groups of physicians have been introduced, and it is clear that the public's access to medical care for Lyme disease is reduced. Individuals are required to take responsibility for finding needed medical care. But the knowledge that this common disease is being so seriously misdiagnosed requires further explanation.

CHAPTER SEVEN

"WHERE ARE THE DOCTORS?"

THE POLITICS OF LYME

I had Lyme disease and was in the hospital because of a 103 degree temperature, very sick and with multiple Lyme rashes. My primary care doctor put me on an intravenous antibiotic. The infectious disease doctor came into my room and ordered the line removed. He said I had already had enough antibiotics for Lyme and was cured of the disease. My doctor then ordered it reinstated, but he received an angry letter from the hospital's infectious disease doctor. He'll keep me as a patient but won't treat me for Lyme. Please help me find a doctor.

—LYME PATIENT WHO HAD BEEN GIVEN FOUR WEEKS OF
DOXYCYCLINE BUT NEEDED FURTHER TREATMENT

Controversy begins with the discovery of the tick bite. Not everyone in the medical community believes in taking preventive antibiotics. Increasingly, however, most people who have either a tick bite or Lyme rash go to their doctors, get a prescription, and have no further problems. It makes no sense to avoid this step, or to wait for a positive test. If symptoms appear or persist beyond a few weeks—or if the disease is not diagnosed in a timely fashion—treatment availability may be less certain. Because of the controversy, few doctors are available to treat disseminated Lyme disease.

Taking an antibiotic can prevent an immune response, and therefore a negative result, if a test is given, does not indicate that the tick did not carry the disease. After a wait of a couple of weeks the (problematic) test might show a positive response, but there is no good reason to wait.

Discovering the Tick Bite and the Controversy

Eugene Shapiro of Yale University, among the authors of both the 2000 and 2006 Infectious Diseases Society of America guidelines, disagrees with giving preventive antibiotics. "It may be reasonable to administer doxycycline in areas where the incidence of Lyme disease is high and when the tick is a nymphal [immature] tick that is partially engorged with blood . . . If chemoprophylaxis is done, only a single dose of doxycycline should be administered."[1] However, there is another point of view: Most knowledgable people consider a single day of treatment an unacceptable risk.

The two sides of the controversy could not be more divided for a disease that poses potential problems. One side says it is easily diagnosed and can be treated in days or weeks. The other says that it can be difficult to identify and treat and should, if possible, be treated until the patient is well.

Allen Steere's 1993 article "The Over Diagnosis of Lyme Disease"[2] divided the medical community. Several doctors challenged this opinion, but Steere's well-known name gave the article greater impact. As late as 1990, Steere acknowledged ongoing neurological Lyme, especially encephalitis (brain disease) and polyneuropathy (peripheral nerve disease) would benefit from antibiotics, but in 1993 he introduced the theory of "post-Lyme syndrome."

"Post-Lyme syndrome" is described as continuing symptoms of Lyme that Steere and his adherents hypothesize are not caused by continuing or chronic Lyme infection but may be the result of a possible autoimmune response or other factors that we do not yet understand. Another cause, as they describe it, may be chronic fatigue syndrome or fibromyalgia. No evidence has been produced for any of these theories. And because there is no treatment, the insurance companies bear no cost. However, a patient's uncertain health status often leads to otherwise unnecessary X-rays, MRIs, and other tests as well as ongoing pain or sleep medications.

Physicians testify for either side of court cases, but the Infectious Diseases Society of America physicians hired by insurance companies have been incredibly effective in denying claims. This seems to be true no matter what the medical history, how severe the illness, or how disabled the patient. In the case of Lyme, IDSA physicians testify against Lyme disease physicians. They deny the patient has Lyme. They also deny that the patient ever had Lyme and may even deny that the patient is sick.

As early as 1996, with the "post-Lyme syndrome" theory in place, Leonard Sigal, an adherent of limiting diagnosis and treatment, testified in the New Jersey Superior Court (case L 2148–94) with regard to *Millar v. Kenny and Glen*. The following is partial testimony with the attorney, Ira Maurer:

Q: Do you have any billing records pertaining to your work in this matter? The last page of the four page document marked as exhibit 4 indicates you had spent eight hours and 40 minutes at a rate of $560 per hour . . .

A: Correct.

[The deposition documents that Dr. Sigal is not trained in infectious disease. He testifies about a contract between his university and a company developing a Lyme disease vaccine and the approximate dollar amount.]

Q: With regard to legal matters, would I be correct that the opinions you've expressed for attorneys has [sic] been either that the diagnosis of Lyme disease is incorrect or that the patient has been over treated?

A: Are you asking is that the sum total of all my opinions?

Q: With regard to opinions you've expressed for attorneys.

A: I suspect that a large percentage of them would be described as you have just stated, but I don't know that I have never stated that somebody, in fact, had Lyme disease . . . in fact, now I think of it there's at least one that comes to mind where I thought the diagnosis had been missed, but the physician did all that was prudent in community standard in looking for the diagnosis of Lyme disease, but I don't believe I have rejected the diagnosis, nor nay say every case [*sic*].

Q: In addition to the work you've done for attorneys, you've also done work for insurance companies. Is that correct?

A: Yes.

[The number of cases in which he is involved is asked, and Dr. Sigal is nonspecific in his answer.]

Q: Would I be correct that the vast majority of the matters you've reviewed for insurance companies have resulted in your expressing opinions that the patient did not have Lyme disease?

A: I—certainly a number of them have led me to believe that the diagnosis of Lyme disease was not documented by the materials I have received.

[Dr. Sigal testified that he had reviewed cases for Prudential, Aetna, Blue Cross/Blue Shield, and other insurance companies that he does not recollect.][3]

THE CONGRESSIONAL HEARING OF 1993

On August 5, 1993, Senator Edward Kennedy, chairman of the Senate Labor and Human Relations Committee, held a congressional hearing to determine the status of Lyme disease research. Personnel from the National Institutes of Health and the Centers for Disease

Control planned the hearing. Speakers included the Yale rheumatologist Allen Steere and a recovered Lyme patient.

Also attending the congressional hearing were patients, researchers, and physicians who believed that Lyme could be a serious disease and asked for representation. Joseph Burrascano of New York, an internist and Lyme disease physician, testified about improprieties that included researchers working as medical consultants for insurance companies. He expressed concern that some of those receiving grants were advocates of the "post-Lyme syndrome" theory, meaning that they held that ongoing symptoms resulted from a condition such as chronic fatigue or fibromyalgia or another unknown illness.

The Congressional hearing was the epochal event that continues to impact physician practice and the lives of Lyme victims today. No action was taken as a result of the hearing, but the division in the world of medicine was laid bare. Despite repeated public requests, Congress held no further hearings on Lyme disease, and it appeared that Congress did not want to address this unexpected response to Lyme disease research.

In 2001, the Lyme disease controversy heated up. The Steere group of physicians appeared ready to address the continuing and increasing opposition to the theory of "post-Lyme syndrome", with the investigation of Dr. Burrascano. The *New York Times Magazine* told the story of the 1993 hearing.

> When Steere arrived to discuss his test results with other experts in the field, the gallery was already packed with spectators . . .
>
> As if to dramatize his allegations, which Steere and other researchers denied, a young boy in a wheelchair appeared. He wore headphones over his ears to block out other voices in the room, which his mother said were deafening due to neurological damage from a Lyme spirochete. As his mother tried to interpret his gestures, the boy leaned forward and whispered into the microphone, "We

can't think," he said of chronic Lyme patients. "We can't sleep. We need you."

The room was aghast. Steere later told a reporter that in his seventeen years of research he had never seen a Lyme case like the boy's. During the Senate discussion he tried to explain why there was so much misdiagnosis in general, but the gallery began to shout, "He's wrong."[4]

THE BURRASCANO CASE

Burrascano's congressional testimony drawing attention to improprieties drew a line in the sand, showing how divergent are the views of physicians who treat Lyme disease and those who don't. Burrascano said,

> There is a core of university-based physicians whose opinions carry a great deal of weight. Unfortunately, many of them act unscientifically and unethically. They adhere to self-serving views and attempt to personally discredit those whose opinions differ from their own. They exert strong, ethically questionable influence on medical journals, which enables them to publish and promote articles that are badly flawed. They work with government agencies to bias the agenda of consensus meetings, and have worked to exclude from these meetings and scientific seminars those with alternate opinions. They behave this way for reasons of personal or professional gain, and are involved in serious conflicts of interest. —Congressional Hearing, Senate Labor and Human Relations Committee, August 5, 1993

In his testimony, Burrascano described how easily Lyme can be acquired with a cost to society measured in billions of dollars (meaning medical costs, job loss, disability, and social costs) and he dismissed the "post-Lyme syndrome" substitution for what is persisting, under-treated disease. He said,

> It is interesting to note that these individuals who pro-mote this "post-Lyme syndrome" as a form of arthritis de-pend on funding from arthritis groups and agencies to earn their livelihood. Some of them are known to have re-ceived large consulting fees from insurance companies to advise them to curtail coverage for any antibiotic therapy beyond this arbitrary 30-day cutoff, even if the patient will suffer. This is despite the fact that additional therapy may be beneficial, and despite the fact that such practices never occur in treating other diseases.
>
> Following the lead of this group of physicians, a few state health departments have even begun to investigate in a very threatening way, physicians who have more lib-eral views on Lyme diagnosis than they do. I must con-fess that I am taking a large personal risk here today by publicly stating these views, despite the fact that many hundreds of physicians and many thousands of patients all over the world would agree with what I am saying here.—Congressional Hearing, Senate Labor and Human Relations Committee, August 5, 1993

Burrascano concluded by describing the missteps in diagnosis, test-ing, and treatment of Lyme disease, saying how the process and the funding were compounding problems and derailing solutions. In ef-fect, he accused Steere and his colleagues of conflict of interest and negligence, with possible legal consequences.

AFTER THE EPOCHAL LYME DISEASE HEARING OF 1993

What followed after the hearing was not the initiation of reasoned sci-entific debate with funds appropriated for long-term, well-controlled research studies that would help determine treatment needs for Lyme disease. What happened instead was that Steere and his colleagues gathered support for their position denying ongoing illness with fundraising and grant proposals that resulted in published articles supporting their view so extensively that in effect it became the standard approach to Lyme disease.

The adherents of limiting treatment for Lyme disease also began harassing attacks on Lyme disease physicians through state medical board contacts. Just two months after his testimony, Dr. Burrascano was notified by the state of New York that he was being investigated for an anonymous complaint against him, though he was not charged at that time.

THE NATOLE CASE

After the Congressional hearing other physicians who treat persisting disease were charged by their state medical boards in regard to Lyme disease treatment. Sometimes the charges were not stated directly using the word *overtreating*, but that was the message. One of them was Joseph Natole, Jr, who came to the attention of Michigan's state medical board by duly reporting all his Lyme cases as required. In 1997 he lost his license to treat Lyme disease for "overtreating" thirty-seven chronic Lyme patients beyond the standard two or three weeks as decided by the Steere adherents. He sought to treat them until they were well, using Burrascano's guidelines, which later became the International Lyme and Associated Diseases Society's guidelines. Allen Steere was one of those testifying against him.[5] There was disbelief that there could be so many cases in Michigan.

In the Circuit Court for the County of Saginaw County in Michigan the Lyme Alliance (a citizen group in Michigan) filed an amicus brief in support of Natole. His appeal was denied on February 10, 1998, with a resulting loss of effective treatment for Lyme disease in Michigan and he was no longer allowed to treat Lyme disease.

According to the Lyme Alliance's newsletter in 2000,

> Dr. Natole diagnosed a patient with Lyme disease, his first
> Lyme case, and the diagnosis was confirmed by a positive
> Lyme test. After seven days of intravenous treatment,
> when the treatment was discontinued, Jane's [the patient]
> health deteriorated and she begged Dr. Natole to contact
> Dr. Burrascano. He contacted the Lyme Disease Founda-
> tion in Connecticut for information, and Dr. Natole was
> put on the referral list. Jane was put back on antibiotics.
>
> This was the beginning of Dr. Natole's involvement in
> treating Lyme disease. Through referrals from the Lyme
> Disease Foundation and word of mouth, his number of
> Lyme patients grew. Dr. Natole began attending Lyme
> conferences and reading all available scientific literature,
> as well as conferring with Dr. Burrascano on a regular ba-
> sis concerning treatment of his Lyme patients. Over a
> five-year period, while his practice rose to over 7,500 pa-
> tients, he saw approximately 2,500 patients for evaluation
> of Lyme disease, diagnosing approximately 250 as having
> chronic Lyme disease.[6]

THE DR. PERRY ORENS CASE

In New York, Dr. Perry Orens lost his license to practice medicine after forty years of unblemished medical practice because he treated his
Lyme patients until they were well. In 1994 a patient of Orens sued
Blue Cross/Blue Shield for denial of payment for intravenous therapy. Testifying against the patient was Raymond Dattwyler, associated
with writing the Infectious Diseases Society of America guidelines,
who said that short-term treatment is the best way to treat Lyme disease. Orens's patient, however, won his case and obtained coverage
for his treatment.

In 1999 Orens's license was revoked by New York's Office of Professional Medical Conduct, the licensing agency for that state. In 2001, the decision was reversed on appeal to the appellate division of the New York Supreme Court. The Office of Professional Medical Conduct then appealed the decision to the next higher court, the Court of Appeals in New York. The vote was 4–3 against Orens.

The Lyme Disease Foundation said in its newsletter (no longer available), "Patients were left with PICC [intravenous] lines in, in the middle of i.v., were left with no treatment and had to have the lines yanked in the emergency room. Children were left without a doctor and deteriorating from lack of treatment as their parents made call after call, only to be turned away."[7]

DR. BURRASCANO OFFICIALLY CHARGED

While the original 1993 complaint against Burrascano was dismissed, the case was kept open. In the summer of 2000, Dr. Burrascano, who had treated more than seven thousand Lyme cases worldwide, was officially charged with medical misconduct. Hearings began in October of that year. Though no patient of Burrascano had ever made a complaint against him, without notice or permission, patient files were removed from his office. Supposedly the selection of charts was random, but all the charts pulled were those of chronic Lyme disease patients.

Before the hearings began, the executive secretary of the Office of Professional Medical Conduct (OPMC) wrote in a letter to a Lyme disease patient, "The Centers for Disease Control, the American Lyme Disease Foundation [founded by Steere supporters]. . . and a host of other sources have provided guidance for the standard of care for Lyme diseases. Rarely, if ever, have these published guidelines indicated anything more than that two or three weeks are required to treat Lyme disease."

However, in another letter responding to a patient who filed a complaint against a doctor who opposed giving him needed longer-term treatment, Dr. Marks, executive secretary of the Office of Professional Medical Conduct, had a different response. "As defined by law, a difference of opinion, in and of itself, is not medical miscon-duct." The Lyme community saw these responses as evidence of bias.

OPMC hearings are secret, and the initial meeting with the tar-geted physician results in no transcript, so the doctor's attorney has no way of subpoenaing the record of this interview. There was no discov-ery process conducted to bring out conflicts of interest (such as which side of the controversy was advocated, insurance or drug company connections, government grants), and the law did not define "expert" for expert witness. Burrascano was not told who the expert was. He was unable to confront his accuser, or know who made the complaint He was also not allowed to discuss what happened in the hearings. It was later determined that the complaint against him most probably came from an insurance company, especially after testimony from the insurance industry at the Albany hearing on November 27, 2001.

Because the debate extends nationwide, Lyme disease organiza-tions and medical boards in other states watched every nuance of the Burrascano trial. Each state has its own procedures for disciplining physicians, and some states investigate physicians who treat Lyme dis-ease, because they are influenced by the same factors as in New York, including the ongoing efforts of IDSA physicians to promote the "post-Lyme syndrome" theory.

Charges can be difficult to defend, regardless of the politics that make Lyme investigations inherently unfair. Ascribing ongoing symp-toms to "post-Lyme syndrome" allows short-term treatment failures to be denied. If this "diagnosis" is made (for which there is no test), patients have no access to treatment. They simply accept that is what they have, a chronic condition, possibly an autoimmune disorder. From then on, they may take other medications, but they will not re-ceive curative treatment. Patients may be deemed either not sick, or the diagnosis has become something other than continuing Lyme.

Success stories occur on an ongoing basis. I see them regularly. Some people are better; some are very much better and have returned to work. Eleanor was in bed for five years with severe muscle weakness, sometimes slurred speech, and memory problems. She recovered completely, with occasional bouts of mild fatigue, and returned to teaching art and traveled to China. Jane, an environmental consultant, who called me regularly for months, was taking oral and then an intravenous antibiotics. She said, "I'm not much better than last month," or, "I think I'm a little better this month," then, "This month I finally drove my car. It's been in the driveway since October." She has since returned to her consulting business, bought a house, and is now well.

These stories of successful outcomes, however, may be characterized by the opposition as "anecdotal" and not "based on evidence." I've heard the opinion expressed, "She probably didn't have Lyme anyway," or "He didn't need all that to get well," or, "It's six months of antibiotics and she's still got symptoms. Doesn't sound to me like it's working."

LYME PATIENTS RALLY

On November 9, 2000, Lyme disease patients held a rally outside the Park Plaza Hotel in New York City. I sat on a stone bench in the park outside the hotel and watched streams of people exiting buses from New York, Connecticut, Michigan, Maine, New Jersey, and Ohio. Two people flew in from California; another came from Florida. Some came with canes and wheelchairs. Four hundred people packed that small square, and, for the first time, I saw others who were sick like me. After the rally, support groups, patients, and patient families launched a campaign to bring the story to an unknowing public. Feared was the loss of still more medical care for Lyme disease victims.

THE *NEW YORK TIMES* BREAKS THE STORY

Six months before the rally and the start of the Burrascano trial, the *New York Times* published a series of articles on the disease. It said what those with chronic Lyme disease had been saying since 1993: We have a potentially serious disease that appears to be poorly diagnosed and inadequately treated.

The *Times* stated,

> Over the past few months, both Dr. Steere and Dr. Burrascano have been ordered by their state's medical boards to answer formal complaints about their practices. Earlier this month, members of Congress from Connecticut, New Jersey and Pennsylvania asked for an inquiry into accusations that federal health officials were using scientific bias and misallocating research money designed for Lyme disease research.

Steere, when interviewed by the reporter Holcomb Noble, said that he "would not comment on individual cases but said that the complaints were 'completely without merit and I am confident they will be dismissed.'" He said he was a victim of "organized harassment," adding that his treatment followed "accepted guidelines."

At the same time, formal complaints of negligence were made to the Massachusetts Board of Registration in Medicine against Allen Steere by seventy-five Lyme patients. The *Times* was able to get copies of some of them. "In recent weeks Dr. Steere has become the subject of seven formal complaints and four letters of complaint filed with the Massachusetts Board of Registration in Medicine by patients who accuse him of misdiagnosing or mistreating their conditions and causing their health to worsen. Copies of their complaints were obtained by the New York Times."

About tests and treatment Steere "agreed that tests done in some laboratories were inaccurate but said that his were not. And on the subject of prolonged antibiotic therapy he said, 'I have been discouraged by what I've seen.' He said he had better success with medications aimed specifically at individual symptoms that persisted, like pain, depression, or chronic fatigue."

In the same article Burrascano spoke of charges that had been filed against him. "Whatever the medical board is saying, what impressed me about all this is that the Lyme patients I see are so incredibly sick. And other doctors are not helping them. I just follow common sense. I listen to my patients and if there's something I can't understand I try to figure it out. I don't just dismiss them."

Without my own Lyme disease experience, I'd have no concept of the importance of the stories published in the *New York Times* and elsewhere. I couldn't have believed that so many people, across the board, would be left untreated or that there could be a possible cover-up. Even the stories of patient suffering would only have bewildered me, and I'd have considered them rare and an anomaly. I would not have believed that patients who continued to be ill would be denied treatment and told they had something else when this answer made no sense.

"THE WAR ON DOCTORS"

The *Times* article quoted Kenneth Liegner, a Lyme specialist in Armonk, New York, as saying that the action taken against Burrascano, "simply amounts to a war on doctors who are just trying to find a way to help patients who are very sick. It's one thing for doctors to want to push their views, but what's going on here is an attempt to stand in the way and prevent others from practicing theirs."[8]

Six months later, following the New York rally, the *Times* said,

> A group of doctors who treat Lyme disease and about 400 patients with the disease accused medical boards in several states of violating doctors rights to treat illness in ways they believe are necessary and scientifically valid. They singled out a current unprofessional conduct hearing against a New York doctor as the latest example.
>
> The doctors and patients reported that about 50 physicians in New York, New Jersey, Connecticut, Michigan, Oregon, Rhode Island and Texas had been investigated, disciplined, or had their licenses removed over the last

three years. This has a chilling effect on the willingness of other doctors to treat the disease, they said.

Speaking at the rally, Michael Schopmann, a lawyer from Lake Success, New York, said that he had represented more than forty doctors in board hearings in New York, New Jersey, and Pennsylvania.

"If a doctor begins to treat Lyme disease in any significant percentage of their total practice," Mr. Schopmann said, "they are guaranteed to face investigation—either private, public or both—by managed care, insurance companies, and state licensing agencies. The treatment of Lyme disease and its financial implications are the insurance industry's worst nightmare."[9]

Several days later, in its article "War Against Doctors," *Newsweek* said that "physicians who use antibiotics aggressively have been scrutinized in Michigan, New Jersey, New York, Pennsylvania, Connecticut, Rhode Island, and Oregon, at the urging of scientists from the other side of the dispute, advocates say. Several have lost their licenses." *Newsweek* said, "The crux of the matter is a seemingly simple technicality—the question of whether or not chronic Lyme consists of chronic infection or persisting symptoms likely fueled by a lingering auto-immune response, originally triggered by the disease. But instead of what should be a cooperative and scholarly quest for the truth, politics, power, and greed have polarized medical professionals, creating what one doctor called an 'all out war.' "[10]

Stephanie Ramp of the *East Hampton Star* wrote of two doctors, Robert Shoen and Eugene Shapiro, who believe the disease is overtreated. She says, "Shoen consults for several insurance companies." And "Shapiro states he has never reviewed individual cases for treatment for insurance companies but has been asked to help formulate the coverage."[11]

Many doctors consult for companies, but, in this controversy, there is no representation from those with a different view of the disease.

Burrascano spoke to the issue of possible dangers of long-term anti-biotics, "You're not going to withhold treatment for a possible side effect, which may never occur, and ignore a known infection that desperately needs to be treated. The reality and truth of Lyme, supported by valid peer-reviewed publications, and our experience with thousands of patients, count for nothing."[12]

In the midst of the Burrascano hearings, those with the opinion that the disease should be treated no more than a few weeks rushed into print with the announcement of soon-to-be-released research studies.[13] Mark Klempner, lead author, and one of the signers of the 2006 IDSA guidelines, concluded from the short-term three-month study of low-dose antibiotics on a limited number of patients (see Chapter 11) that there was no benefit in long-term treatment. In his published research before 1993, Klempner did acknowledge possible long-term Lyme, as did Steere, who also wrote of possible long-term neurological problems, but both have since changed their views of the disease to describe ongoing illness as "post-Lyme syndrome."

Shortly after the studies were published in the *New England Journal of Medicine*, they were given wide newspaper and medical journal publicity. They've also been used ever since by insurance companies who limit coverage for Lyme disease treatment.

Sam Donta commented that these should be the first of a series of studies, and questioned why the study was designed to test only one course of antibiotics. The chosen antibiotics, Rocephin or doxycycline, were given for a designated amount of time, with no re-treatment. Donta said, regarding the studies, that the antibiotics were not given for a long enough time, and he would have chosen different ones. Perhaps all the studies show, he said, is "that this particular treatment doesn't work."[14]

Of the approximately dozen physicians who actively oppose continuing treatment for Lyme, several commented in the *Times*, supporting the Klempner conclusions. Within the next two or three years, these physicians published more studies, including one by Gary Wormser, who concluded that ten days of treatment might be sufficient.

Allen Steere was then at the New England Medical Center and did not comment—he's now at the Massachusetts General Hospital and professor of medicine at Harvard University. He no longer spoke to reporters after the June 17 *New York Times* article. Grann reported on the difficulty of setting up an appointment with Steere, saying, "Things had gotten so bad that by the time I reached Steere in February [for the June 17 article] he had gone into seclusion, refusing to give interviews, and, according to a friend, traveling to speaking engagements under an alias." The publicist from the public relations firm that Steere had hired told Grann, "He's worried that any publicity will make him more of a target."

I recalled my experience seven years earlier, at the Steere-run Lyme disease clinic, when the physicians on duty told me I didn't have Lyme and dismissed me with a "cheery good luck."

BURRASCANO EXONERATED

After a year of investigation, on November 8, 2001, Dr. Burrascano was exonerated of most of the thirty-nine charges brought against him. Isolated findings of guilt would not prevent him from continuing to practice or to treat Lyme disease according to his best judgment. These are excerpts from the board's decision:

> The Hearing Committee recognizes the existence of the current debate within the medical community over issues concerning management of patients with recurrent or long-term disease. This appears to be a highly polarized and politicized conflict as was demonstrated to this committee by expert testimony from both sides, each supported by numerous medical journal articles, and participants each emphatic that the opposition position was clearly incorrect.

What clearly did emerge, however, was that the Respon-
dent's approach, while certainly a minority viewpoint, is one
that is shared by many other physicians. We recognize that
the practice of medicine may not always be an exact science,
"issued guidelines" are not regulatory and patient care is frequently individualized.

Lyme disease organizations, volunteers, and Lyme patients next set
their sights on reforming New York's Office of Professional Medical
Conduct. In January 2002, two months after the Albany hearing on
chronic Lyme disease, a hearing was held in Manhattan with the focus on
needed changes in the OPMC. On April 17, 2002, the New York Legislature Assembly Health Committee passed a resolution on the treatment of doctors by the Office of Professional Medical Conduct. It
acknowledged the legitimacy of Lyme disease treatment and the involvement of insurance companies in targeting doctors. It asked OPMC to
"cease and desist" from targeting those who treat Lyme disease.

Three years later, on June 15, 2005, the Director of the Office of
Professional Medical Conduct, Dennis Graziano, issued a memorandum that was copied to all staff members, and sent to board members of the Board of the Office of Professional Medical Conduct
and its chief counsel. "This memorandum is intended to memorial-
ize and endorse the principles that are currently in place . . . regarding investigation of physicians, physician assistants, and specialists
who use treatment modalities not universally accepted by the medical profession, such as the varying treatment modalities of the Lyme
disease and other tick-borne diseases." Further, the memorandum
says, "so long as a treatment modality effectively treats legitimate
disease, pain, injury, deformity of physical condition, the recommendation of this modality does not, by itself, constitute professional
misconduct."

This was a win for Dr. Burrascano, for the Lyme community, and for those who will need treatment in the future, but it did not guarantee that charges could not be brought again in some other way, or that New York physicians who treat Lyme disease are protected as well as they might be. And each state operates by its own rules, so this did not protect physicians nationwide.

Thousands of Lyme patients from across the country had bombarded legislators, the attorney general, and the governor of New York with letters and telephone calls. The Burrascano victory and the reforms in New York did not solve problems for all those with Lyme disease. Other state medical boards are influenced by the controversy over Lyme disease. They have long received pressure from insurance companies and their consultants to muzzle the Lyme problem, and this continues to occur. In other states, too, the legal process may be secretive and flawed, and insurance claims denied. Judges may see the Lyme debate as a medical issue that they are not qualified to decide. They defer to experts, and the experts can be expected to represent one single point of view, that of the Infectious Diseases Society of America. Therefore, in most court cases and licensing hearings, without major effort and support from knowledgeable people, neither the patient nor the doctor can expect to prevail.

When physicians are investigated, the charge may not be that they are overdiagnosing or overtreating Lyme, rather it is likely to be indirect, such as a procedural error, a problem with a record, or not monitoring the patient sufficiently. But the testimony is about Lyme, diagnosing too much and challenging the need for antibiotic treatment. Physicians who practice alternative medicine are not investigated, nor are physicians who give long-term treatment, even if unproven, for other conditions such as arthritis, depression, or high cholesterol. They are not questioned in the same way. Nor are antibiotics limited for other condition such as tuberculosis, malaria, or even the skin condition of acne. For Lyme, it's different, and only antibiotics can be expected to cure Lyme disease.

PEOPLE MAGAZINE

Opposition to diagnosing and treating persistent Lyme has not gone away, and politics help ensure that physicians still do not receive adequate information when seeing patients who may have Lyme. The IDSA has unusually good access to medical journals and texts and continues to promote its standard of care. In 2003, *People* magazine described the "hidden plague," telling the story of the devastation that may result from it. A young man, seriously ill with undiagnosed Lyme, was rushed to an emergency room, where he was told that he had Lou Gehrig's disease, likely to kill him in six months. He was hooked to a feeding tube. A relative considered another possible cause of his illness and suggested that he see Dr. Gregory Bach who treats Lyme disease. A bull's-eye rash was found beneath the man's hair. He rebounded after he was treated with antibiotics, remained on the antibiotic for fourteen months, and was cured. "Lyme is a much more serious disease than the public recognizes," said Brian Fallon of Columbia University's Lyme & Tick-borne Diseases Research Center. "People can have cognitive problems for the rest of their lives."[15]

YANKEE MAGAZINE

It's no surprise that medical care for the Lyme disease epidemic is hard to find. In 2007, in *Yankee* magazine, Edie Clark explained the Lyme disease controversy and described what happened to a New Hampshire woman. "The day before I got sick, I ran 10 miles, played nine holes of golf, and then I painted the living room. That was my typical day." The next day she was sick. "I was so tired, like nothing I remember in my life; I just wanted to sleep. I dragged myself to work, got through the day, and came home and slept and slept. And I was freezing. It was a hot day, and I crawled into a sleeping bag and curled up in a chair shivering." She consulted approximately fifteen to twenty doctors, including doctors at Boston's Lahey Clinic and Beth Israel Deaconess Medical Center, and was diagnosed with chronic fatigue syndrome, Crohn's disease, anorexia, depression, and empty nest syndrome. She found a Lyme doctor, went on a year and a half of antibiotics, and is now nearly well.[16]

LYME ACTIVISTS FIGHT BACK

As early as 1999, before the Burrascano trial, the public became involved in political action to allow treatment for Lyme disease. The *Boston Globe* said, "A renowned Boston doctor who is credited with naming the disease in 1978 is expected to run into a hostile group of patients when he gives a talk on the illness today at the National Institutes of Health. . . . Protestors say Steere's guidelines are obsolete, biologically unfounded, and ethically suspect."[17]

TWO POINTS OF VIEW IN MEDICAL TEXT

In the 1997 edition of *Conn's Current Therapy*, the classic textbook for physicians, Joseph Burrascano wrote the section on methods of diagnosing and treating Lyme disease. In the 1998 edition this section was written by Allen Steere, with information very different from that published in the 1997 edition. Burrascano wrote of possible difficulty in treating Lyme disease and need for individualized, and often extensive, care. On the other hand, Steere presented his standard of care supported by the IDSA physicians who limit treatment to low-dose antibiotics for less than four weeks.

In 1999, the year preceding the Burrascano trial, the Connecticut attorney general, Richard Blumenthal, convened a public hearing on insurance coverage for Lyme disease. A bill was being developed to mandate Connecticut health insurance companies to pay for long-term intravenous antibiotic therapy for children and adults with Lyme. The hearing was arranged to contrast the two points of view on the disease. Two representatives, for example, from Connecticut's largest insurance companies said it was their general policy to pay for a maximum of six weeks for intravenous therapy for Lyme disease but said they would, however, pay for prolonged oral therapy. Two patients gave testimony about their Lyme experiences and what they had suffered.

Two physicians also testified for the Burrascano viewpoint. Among their many comments, Steven Phillips and Amiram Katz spoke of chronic disease that occurs without positive blood tests. On the other side, Robert Shoen and Matthew Cartter then spoke for the over-diagnosed, overtreated side on the dangers of overtreatment. Dr. Cartter was the petitioner in 2007 for proposed changes made by the Council of State and Territorial Epidemiologists that would narrow the criteria for reporting Lyme disease.

In June 1999, the Connecticut legislature passed Public Act 99–2, which mandates health insurance companies to pay for not fewer than thirty days of intravenous antibiotic therapy for children and adults with presumed Lyme disease. Objective findings and/or positive B. burgdorferi serology (blood tests) are not required. In addition, insurance companies are mandated to pay for more than thirty days of intravenous antibiotic therapy ordered in consultation with a board-certified rheumatologist, neurologist, or infectious disease specialist. Again objective findings and/or positive B. burgdorferi serology is not required.

This was the first Lyme legislation to be passed. Besides Connecticut, several other states have taken legislative action to assure medical treatment coverage and protection of physicians who treat Lyme disease. Those requiring medical care who are having insurance problems may need to know what legislative relief may be available in their states.

In Rhode Island, on July 7, 2002, Governor Donald Carcieri signed into law the Lyme Disease Diagnosis and Treatment Act, which had been passed on July 2. It had strong support, assisted by the work of the Rhode Island Chapter of the Lyme Disease Association. It mandates coverage by insurance companies that are licensed in Rhode Island for physician-prescribed Lyme disease treatment when ordered by a treating physician who deems it necessary.

The California Lyme Disease Association (CALDA) is one of the most active Lyme disease associations and publishes the *Lyme Times* to inform patients and physicians on aspects of the disease. CALDA was instrumental in getting bill AB 592 into law on September 22, 2005. The legislation says that physicians may not be disciplined solely for alternative or complementary treatments. The California law originated from the New York policy memorandum on the Office of Professional Medical Conduct.

In Maryland, Lyme activists opposed the IDSA's efforts to disseminate its guidelines to Maryland physicians. In New Jersey, two bills were passed on curriculum guidelines for schools and teacher education. Florida Lyme patients have been successful in introducing bills to mandate insurance coverage for long-term antibiotics and other therapies as deemed medically necessary.

Massachusetts has introduced comprehensive legislation on Lyme disease education, medical coverage, and protection of physicians who treat the disease. The Massachusetts Department of Public Health sponsors a Lyme and other tick-borne diseases task force, led by Alfred DeMaria, chief medical officer of the department, and Bela Matyas, medical director of the epidemiology program. It includes physician representatives from both sides of the controversy, but its mandate does not include addressing the Lyme debate.

"THE STANDARD OF CARE RULE"

In the middle 1980s, the decision was made to put AIDS research in the infectious disease branch of the National Institutes of Health (NIH). Lyme disease research, that of another emerging infection, was placed in the arthritis and immunology part of NIH, which may have had to do with Allen Steere's being a rheumatologist. In the opinion of many, some of the Lyme research problems derive from the fact that Lyme, an infectious disease, is not located in the infectious diseases part of NIH, making more likely the autoimmune hypotheses. In autoimmune diseases, the body's immune system fails to recognize its own body parts, and an aberrant response results in destruction of its own cells and tissues. This occurs, for example, in lupus and rheumatoid arthritis.

All manner of Lyme research is done on many aspects of Lyme disease. Those with strong ties to the National Institutes of Health receive grants for the nature of possible "post-Lyme syndrome," autoimmune disease, whether multiple sclerosis could be triggered by Lyme (or should the diagnosis have been Lyme?), whether there is a genetic factor that triggers Lyme "arthritis." Research studies, however, with the exception of the problematic Klempner study, have largely, with the exception of the Fallon study, avoided the needed evidence-based, long-term, double-blinded treatment study that is needed for chronic Lyme disease.

Arrayed against the all-important focus of finding the most effective treatment for Lyme disease is a formidable power structure that in 2000 had been in place for seven years, continuing to grow, largely working unnoticed and unchallenged, spreading its influence to almost every part of the medical care system. Experience and evidence to the contrary has been either ignored, or other explanations are found. Challengers with a different point of view become marginalized. The campaign most visible to the public was the case against Joseph Burrascano.

The question is asked frequently, "Why are those who don't diagnose or treat Lyme disease beyond the initial weeks not held accountable?" The "standard of care rule" that the overdiagnosed side of the controversy seeks to impose for Lyme disease provides the basis for attacking physicians and denying insurance claims.

For Lyme and other medical conditions, however, "the standard of care rule" means that physicians who follow "standard practice," that is, if they do generally what other physicians do, are usually protected against investigation and lawsuits, even if the treatment is later proved wrong. For other conditions—whether pneumonia, hepatitis, malaria, and so on—physicians usually have choices and treatment options. But not for Lyme. In place has been the short-term treatment protocol, and because many physicians know no other, many have come to see it as the standard of care for Lyme disease.

The standard of care holds, even when what physicians do is not based on objective, scientific evidence. Often, cases that are described in medical journals appear as no more than anecdotal, or published reports describe only a limited number of cases. Treatments may change, but if physicians follow the "standard practice" of their time they are usually trouble free. "We didn't have the studies," they can say. "We didn't know."

As a result, those who limit diagnosis and treatment of Lyme disease have been virtually unaccountable, even if patients make ongoing trips to emergency rooms or end up in wheelchairs. Insurance companies pay for "something else," such as drugs for fibromyalgia or chronic fatigue symptoms, but they are not paying for Lyme. Because those in power have worked to make limited treatment "standard practice," they have been able to become nearly unaccountable for what would otherwise be deemed negligence. They are following "standards of care." But they are the ones who wrote them.

When seventy-five seriously ill patients filed complaints against Allen Steere, there was no way he could be made accountable because he was simply doing what other physicians do regarding medical care for Lyme disease. Those defending the overdiagnosed, overtreated side can safely say, as they do now, "He didn't have Lyme and he doesn't have Lyme now, but we treated him (short-term) anyway just in case. We don't know why he has continuing symptoms. Maybe he has an autoimmune disease. We need more studies." The other side says, "Let's stay with the treatment."

The cure for all Lyme can't be found in short-term antibiotic care. So the search must continue, using long-term care in the meantime, since researchers have not figured out the appropriate methods.

It is ironic that physicians whose goal is to treat until well—and care for the needs of those desperately ill—find themselves under attack, not by their patients but by other physicians. For those in power, the solution to dissent has been to try to eliminate physicians espousing a different view, and perhaps also the risk of a class action suit by wronged patients.

"THE REASONABLE MAN RULE"

In addition to the standard of care rule, there is the "reasonable man" rule, saying that a physician may do what a prudent man would do under similar circumstances, using his best judgment and knowledge. One might ask, "How can a prudent physician with sick patients justify limiting treatment to four weeks, watching patients remain ill, and saying, with no proof whatsoever, that they no longer have Lyme disease?" But because the apparent intent of the physician investigations appears to be that of eliminating opposition, opportunities for defense have been limited. The purpose does not appear as that of providing a fair playing field.

With most of the Lyme disease funding and resources going to the IDSA physicians, there is inequity of resources between the two sides. The IDSA has the ear of the CDC and the National Institutes of Health. The result is that needs of patients have been virtually ignored. The crucial long-term treatment study is not yet done, allowing unproven theories to halt progress in our ability to treat and cure Lyme disease.

"WHY DON'T PHYSICIANS KNOW WHAT CAN HAPPEN TO PEOPLE WHO GET LYME DISEASE?"

Because undiagnosed, untreated, and undertreated patients usually go away, as I did, taking their symptoms elsewhere, physicians may never know the outcome of their decisions and are under no obligation to follow up on patients. Those who are undiagnosed or misdiagnosed and go to other doctors seldom provide feedback to their former physicians. A report received may be viewed as interesting, but "anecdotal." As well, because Lyme is a multisystem disease, crossing the lines of several specialties depending on the symptoms presented, a single case may involve many doctors. Patients, especially if they are not diagnosed and successfully treated, visit physicians specializing in neurology, gastroenterology, rheumatology, ophthalmology, cardiology, and psychiatry, none of whom may know about Lyme disease as a possible cause.

As a general rule, physicians are not accountable for missed or incorrect diagnoses, ineffective treatment, or treatment with a bad outcome. Courts are outcome oriented, and an obviously harmful result must be demonstrated for patients to win a case. No harm may be apparent from not diagnosing or treating Lyme disease, so patients cannot easily sue for negligence.

PATIENTS' RIGHTS

"If you don't know you have rights, you don't have them." Patients have the right to refuse treatment—they also have the right to choose treatment. Under the ethical principle of autonomy, the treatment decision belongs to the patient, with risk, benefits, and alternate treatment information provided by physicians. Patients also have the right to view and receive copies of their medical records, change doctors, and get second opinions. Patients don't have the right to receive treatment. Ultimately, the physician's decision to deny treatment stands, right or wrong, politically motivated or not. Currently, going to another physician without experience with Lyme disease is unlikely to help those with persisting disease, because the "standard of care" now in place reflects the views of those who deny chronic Lyme disease.

With the advent of managed care, patients have lost, to some degree, the rights of the marketplace. Treatment choices have narrowed to fit the current health care model where medical treatment decisions are often made by insurance companies. Especially with an uncertain disease like Lyme, enrollment in a health maintenance plan may not be the best choice.

LEGAL RIGHTS FOR NEGLIGENCE AND MISDIAGNOSIS

Those who know the Lyme treatment story ask why patients who face the results of neglect and the misdiagnosis of Alzheimer's or multiple sclerosis don't complain to their state medical boards or join a class action suit, as occurred with the Lymerix vaccine. They can indeed do this, whether or not it results in discipline of the doctor who did not treat their disease. If enough complaints are filed, boards become educated and doctors are more likely to be protected against investigations for treating chronic Lyme. In addition, there are several U.S. lawyers with wide experience in sheltering physicians against unwarranted intrusions by politically connected medical boards.

HOW TO GET LYME DISEASE TREATMENT

Medical care for Lyme disease can be found. It is available. Patients can bring information to physicians and make known their wishes not to take chances with their health. Preventive antibiotics are becoming increasingly available, as has longer-term treatment—with knowledge of the spreading tick problem.

At least one, two, or three antibiotic refills, each one usually lasting a month, may be available. If someone becomes ill, and doesn't respond to initial treatment, the physician can consult with one of the leading physicians experienced in treating the persisting disease. Physicians treating Lyme disease may use not just one treatment regimen. As they do for other diseases, they will use those with which they have had the most success. Other health care providers, including nurse practitioners, who have attended meetings and conferences that have alerted them to the Lyme treatment problem, may also address the potential seriousness of this illness.

After understanding the issues, most people can find the help they need to prevent the disease from becoming chronic. If it has already become entrenched, it can be treated as well. The Lyme Disease Association, the International Lyme and Associated Diseases

Society, and the Lyme Disease Foundation all provide information and resources. In many states, there are chapters and local support groups that provide telephone numbers and people to call. Check the listed Web sites in the Resources section of this book for the latest information.

CHAPTER EIGHT

"WILL I EVER GET WELL?"

TREATING PERSISTENT LYME DISEASE
THE JARISCH-HERXHEIMER REACTION

*There has never in the history of this illness been one study that proves even
in the simplest way that 30 days of antibiotic therapy cures Lyme disease.
However, there is a plethora of documentation in the US and European literature demonstrating histologically and in culture that short courses of
antibiotic treatment fail to eradicate the Lyme spirochete.*
—INTERNATIONAL LYME AND ASSOCIATED DISEASES SOCIETY

As has been emphasized throughout this book, obstacles inherent
in our medical care system may prevent early and adequate
treatment of Lyme disease. Lack of information increases the likeli-
hood of contracting difficult-to-treat Lyme. By understanding the
politics and knowing the hurdles that Lyme patients commonly face,
you can make sure you receive the care you may need. This chapter
tells you about antibiotics that are used. It informs you of the possible
Jarisch-Herxheimer response to antibiotics, and how it can, unnecessarily, derail treatment. I tell about my experience with this reaction
and describe ways that I coped with the disease.

BE PREPARED

- If you discover an attached tick, observe a rash, and receive a positive test result, you can expect to be given the standard (antibiotic) doxycycline prescription of two pills a day for two to four weeks. The dose given may be higher, perhaps three pills per day.
- For a known tick bite but no rash and positive test result, the physician will likely also give doxycycline as a preventive antibiotic. It may depend on information that the doctor has been given and the request made by the patient.

Doxycycline, an antibiotic in the tetracycline family, is used for many conditions, including acne, urinary tract infections, and gum disease, as well as for people who may have been exposed to anthrax. Like tetracycline, it is not used for pregnant women or for children under eight because of possible tooth discoloration in developing teeth. It is taken with food to avoid possible stomach discomfort, but neither it nor tetracycline can be taken with milk because calcium diminishes its effectiveness. Other antibiotics, as described in the International and Associated Diseases Society treatment guidelines, may be used.

- Possible Lyme symptoms without a known tick bite presents the biggest challenge of all. If symptoms appear that don't resolve, such as headache or flulike illness, but there is neither a rash nor a positive test, some doctors give antibiotics. Many, however, don't, because they do not have supportive information, such as known tick exposure, that connects the symptoms with the need for an antibiotic. And, after symptoms develop, they no longer see antibiotics as preventive, with the comment, "There is no proof that this is Lyme."

The Time Factor

Time may be required to get a medical appointment, and preventive treatment can be therefore delayed. If you find a tick and remove it, as described earlier and in pamphlets on tick removal, it is wise to save the tick. If you don't save it, the doctor takes your word that you were bitten and provides the preventive antibiotic.

If you are on vacation, and seek a doctor to prescribe a preventive antibiotic, getting more than a one-day prescription is sometimes difficult, regardless of the presence of a rash. Robert Nadelman of the Infectious Diseases Society of American advocated a single dose of doxycycline for preventing Lyme disease in his 2001 article in the *New England Journal of Medicine*[1] and his position has not changed. Save the tick and ask for a preventive antibiotic, requesting that the duration be at least a week.

Keep in mind that the IDSA guidelines, and the associated medical literature, give the message to doctors that a physician-documented rash of five centimeters is required. Rashes, however, often take time to develop, if they appear at all, and there is no standard size. In addition, doctors have been also told that a single dose of antibiotic may be sufficient treatment (to prevent infection). Especially if the tick was not discovered soon after it became attached, this may be a completely fallacious judgment.

Going to the emergency room is a possibility but unlikely to be more helpful. The tick will be removed, though, and its presence will be documented in the medical record. Many people use this option because they are unsure how to remove the tick correctly and prefer to have someone else do it. The standard procedure is that an emergency room doctor or nurse removes the tick, gives a one-day, hopefully at least a several-day, dose of doxycycline, and refers the patient to his or her physician for follow-up. The emergency room is an expensive way to deal with a tick bite.

What Should Happen

Scott noticed a red spot on his arm during the days following an afternoon of yard work. Upon examining the spot more closely, it appeared to be a tick. At the hospital emergency room the doctor removed it but Scott was given just two pills. He asked for more and was refused. However, he had access to a Lyme-literate physician and was given a one-week supply of doxycycline. The tick was sent to a laboratory for testing. The negative result came back in a week, the antibiotic was stopped, and unless he gets another tick bite, he has no further concern about having contracted a potentially serious spirochetal infection from an afternoon of yard work.

Our medical system does not, for most people, provide the service for the testing of ticks, and people pursue this option on their own. Unlike the ELISA or Western blot tests that are given to people, ticks can be tested and the results are reliable. Without testing the tick, you can have no assurance that the tick does not carry Lyme disease and that "it was only attached for a short time." The percentage of ticks carrying Lyme disease is high, well over 50 percent in some counties in the Northeast and upper midwestern areas of the country. In many states the percentage of infected ticks has not yet been researched, but we already know that the number of infected ticks continues to increase everywhere, and that Lyme disease has spread across the United States. You cannot assume that the tick was not infected.

Keeping Your Own Supply of Antibiotic

"I garden and pull off a tick, sometimes several, and can't keep going to the doctor for every tick bite. He has been treating our family for years and we keep a bottle [of doxycycline] on hand." Some people with frequent tick exposure keep a supply handy, but most don't have access to this possibility, since doxycycline is an antibiotic requiring prescription by a doctor or nurse practitioner.

THE AMERICAN ACADEMY OF PEDIATRICS (APA) AND LYME DISEASE

Not only do the IDSA and the American Neurology Association rec-ommend against preventive treatment, so does the American Academy of Pediatrics. It is contrary to what I, and all who seek adequate med-ical care for Lyme disease, believe. It says in its policy statement on its website, "Routine use of antibiotics to prevent Lyme disease after a deer tick bite is not recommended, even in endemic areas." About testing, the statement says,

> Serologic [blood] testing at the time of a recognized tick bite is not recommended. There is little or no chance that a patient would have detectable antibodies to Borrelia burgdorferi from a new infection at the time of a tick bite and antibodies present would likely represent a false-positive [sic] result or evidence of an earlier infection. Although some physicians obtain a serum sample 6 to 8 weeks later for antibody testing to provide reassurance in the absence of an erythema migrans rash or antibiotic therapy, this practice is unusually unnecessary, especially with evidence that the tick was attached for 48 hours, and the result may be misleading because of the inaccuracy of serological testing for Lyme disease in many laboratories. There is a high probability of false-positive [sic] serologic test result for Lyme disease when the probability of the presence of Lyme disease is low.

This recommendation indicates that parents of children who are bitten by deer ticks need do nothing. Regarding testing, false posi-tives are mentioned, but not false negatives, although the ILADS states that false negatives are more often the problem. Not even a single dose of preventive antibiotic is included in the American Academy of Pediatrics statement. It says that the risk of infection is low and mentions the possibility of an adverse reaction to a preventive antibiotic.

It sees risk in terms of cost-benefit, as do insurance companies, rather than in terms of protecting the health of children. There will be those who are bitten by an uninfected tick, and the possibility of disease is not viewed as high enough to warrant the costs of preventive treatment. Not recognized are the risks and costs of chronic illness. Parents need to be aware that APA recommendations are made on this basis, as are those of the American Neurological Assocation and the Infectious Diseases Society of America. They do not guarantee that your children are protected from the risk of Lyme disease.

The Myths About Lyme Disease

The public is frequently given well-meant misinformation. For example, with increasing numbers of ticks and news reports on the Lyme disease problem, a community group asked for a physician speaker on Lyme disease. The lecturer, a recently trained internist who practices in a major hospital, made all of the following statements, and none of them are true.

- "If the body of the tick is removed, the tick will expel on its own."
- "Ninety percent of those bitten will have a rash."
- "If it's Lyme disease the center portion of the rash will clear."
- "The Lyme rash lasts a week."
- "Only a small number of ticks transmits Lyme disease."
- "With neurological symptoms, a spinal tap will diagnose the disease."
- "Disseminated disease requires intravenous therapy of four weeks."
- "It takes forty-eight hours for a tick to attach."

From information in preceding pages, it is clear that these are myths. Unsubstantiated statements are commonly made about ticks and Lyme disease, many of them giving false reassurance.

After the Preventive Antibiotic

No answer can be given about how long to take the antibiotic. It is a matter of how much risk is acceptable in regard to the possibility of acquiring disease. A biologist who works in tick-filled woods says, "I wouldn't accept less than six weeks." There is also no way to know whether you have been given enough antibiotic to prevent future problems. If vertigo, muscle pain, or other symptoms occur later, will they be connected to the tick bite you had a couple of months ago? No research has been done, as is the case with other aspects of the disease. We don't know how long the antibiotic should be taken, and each case is different. But if symptoms develop, there is no logic in stopping treatment, and if symptoms reappear later, ask for re-treatment.

For example, my rash occurred six months after my second tick bite. Symptoms appeared quickly after the dried-up tick was removed from under my skin. I was given only two weeks of doxycycline. At my insistence, I was given two more weeks, but my disease continued to worsen over the following weeks and months. The low-dose short-term antibiotic was all but useless. My Lyme infection had been festering without symptoms for six months.

And this was my second bite. It is possible that I may have had more bites that I didn't know about. Among factors affecting the course of Lyme may be how much infection is present, the strain of the Borrelia burgdorferi spirochete, whether or not coinfections are present, how long the tick was attached, and other factors that are unknown.

As there is no definitive time the tick must be attached to transmit disease, there is also no certain length of time that antibiotics may be required, or how high the dose should be. There can be no "standard," and doxycycline is only one of the antibiotics that may be used for treating the disease besides tetracycline, clarithromycin, and others.

High-dose amoxicillin is sometimes given, especially for pregnant women. See the ILADS treatment guidelines.

• If, at the end of a few weeks, following a tick bite, you have symptoms such as flu, fatigue, pain, numbness, dizziness, ask for more treatment. Don't wait for symptoms to "go away." If symptoms subside then recur, keep asking for the antibiotics. Because most physicians, even in highly endemic areas, are not accustomed to treating long-term Lyme disease, which does not resolve in a few weeks, you may need to seek a specialist who treats persisting Lyme. The responsibility is the patient's.

• In case you need to be treated for Lyme disease that is no longer in the blood and has entered body tissues and the brain, and therefore is not easily accessible to antibiotics, ask questions at the first visit. If you develop symptoms after the preventive antibiotic, or they continue after treatment, ask further questions. Will refills be given, and under what circumstances? How much flexibility in regard to duration and antibiotic choice can you expect? Is your physician or nurse practitioner willing to consider other antibiotics beyond doxycycline if your condition appears to require this? Say it is important to know, because if you do have the disease, research studies support frequent need for longer treatment, as documented by the Lyme organizations. Say that the controversy over Lyme disease has resulted in denying adequate treatment for many who need it, and you don't want to risk becoming a victim.

• Even without a known exposure to ticks, if you are ill with what might be symptoms of Lyme disease, for example, continuing fatigue, unexplained pain, and a pattern of symptoms that seems to make no sense, you could have been exposed, either in the outdoors, or by a pet that may have brought a tick into the house. Consider the possibility of Lyme. Cases of flu do not persist for weeks or months. If the cause of your illness remains unknown, and other illnesses, such as arthritis or MS, have been ruled out, ask for a course of antibiotics, whatever the Lyme test results show, and whether or not you recall a tick bite. Don't accept, "It can't be Lyme." All too often people are diagnosed years after receiving many misdiagnoses.

EARLY TREATMENT

Karen found an attached deer tick and removed it. At my urging, she went to her doctor and asked for two weeks of doxycycline. She developed a painful knee, and I suggested that she ask for a refill. Her doctor was unsure that her knee problem was related to Lyme and was reluctant to prescribe, saying, "You shouldn't take too many antibiotics." Karen's knee joint continued to worsen. It began to swell, and she found it hard to walk. Fearing that the disease might progress, and she would be unable to receive care, she returned without an appointment and limped from the parking lot to the office. She remained in the waiting room until she was seen. The doctor then disappeared for about twenty minutes, perhaps seeking further information and, when he returned, gave a refill of three weeks. With another visit, Karen was able to get one more week for a total of six weeks. By that time, her symptoms resolved, and she has had no further problems. "If I hadn't gone to the doctor for the antibiotic, I would have accepted that I had arthritis and my life would have been very different. My doctor already had me lined up with a rheumatologist."

Anita's husband noticed a large pink area across the back of her shoulder. He knew about my case and asked if it could be Lyme. Anita was tested, and the result was positive. She said she felt tired and "achy." With the positive test, she had no problem getting two weeks of antibiotic. She said she still felt "lousy" though. I asked what she was going to do next. Her doctor refused more antibiotic, suggesting that she had chronic fatigue. At my urging, she pursued further treatment, going to another doctor who gave her a total of eight weeks of treatment. There is no way to know whether that was long enough to prevent future problems, but her achiness disappeared, as did her rash.

In my experience, eight to ten weeks has been about the maximum amount of treatment that most people can expect to receive unless they find a doctor who understands the controversy and is knowledge-able about treating Lyme disease. Cost cutting in the health care indus-try is the priority and hinders physician ability to treat this disease. Only public awareness of the Lyme problem can change the response to a Lyme infection.

While many people pursue treatment after a tick bite, others, even with painful symptoms that could be caused by Lyme, prefer to do nothing more. "I don't want to think about Lyme. It could be Lyme, but I get along okay." "My doctor says there's no need." "I don't like to take antibiotics. I'll wait and see if I get better on my own." "I have chronic fatigue syndrome." On the other hand, hundreds of patients regularly travel out of state for Lyme disease care, many paying out of pocket for long-neglected and misdiagnosed disease.

TREATING LYME DISEASE MAY REQUIRE PERSISTENCE

Because symptoms are often variable and intermittent, progress may not be as evident as one might expect. Considerable time is often re-quired before symptoms disappear, or become milder and less fre-quent. Those who don't know the story may give up treatment, saying that "it doesn't work," or "I've had treatment and my doctor says my problem is fibromyalgia."

A friend told me, "My daughter is a pharmacist, and she says if an an-tibiotic doesn't work in three months, it's not effective." Another friend told me, "I had pneumonia and was only treated for three weeks." At a routine medical visit, after reading my history, the doctor said, "You aren't still being treated for Lyme? Your symptoms can't still be Lyme. You need to go to Dr. Steere's Lyme disease clinic. I'll get you an ap-pointment." Even months later, my diagnosis was questioned because I hadn't recovered from the disease in a few weeks.

A major problem for those with a Lyme rash, and symptoms as well, is seeing a doctor promptly for early treatment. It may take a while to get an appointment, and it's unclear whether or not you will be given adequate doxycycline or other antibiotics. Many find themselves in this difficult situation, and there's often no clear answer. With worsening signs of illness, it may take weeks or months to see a physician who treats disease that does not resolve in two weeks, so people must be persistent and do as they can.

It's a good idea to take a picture of the rash, if you have one, and to bring a copy of this book to your doctor. The rash lasts an uncertain amount of time, but that is not the determining factor. You don't want to be shortchanged on preventive or early treatment, and it's unclear on how long you can wait without consequences. Try to avoid this risk in every way you can.

Effective treatment requires a partnership between patient and physician. There is no guarantee that you can prevent it from developing, and you cannot know when all spirochetes may have been eradicated. But it's only common sense that taking antibiotics promptly after a tick bite offers you the best chance for success.

ANTIBIOTICS USED FOR TREATING LYME DISEASE

Doxycycline has been the standard antibiotic for prevention and for early disease, but is not the only one. Others include Biaxin, which is used for a number of bacterial diseases, and tetracycline. Sam Donta finds tetracycline effective in treating Lyme disease, and it was in my case.

You and your doctor may consult the International Lyme and Associated Diseases Society guidelines for information about antibiotics. Joseph Burrascano's thirty-page "Diagnostic Hints and Treatment Guidelines for Lyme and Other Tick-Borne Illnesses" contains information and treatment protocols and is available from the ILADS.

Often, more than one antibiotic is used at the same time in combination, and dosages may be higher than those used for other more easily treated infections. Treatment is not the same for everyone, especially if the disease has become chronic. There is no defining point when it can be considered chronic, but when progress is slow and it is difficult to treat, taking prolonged amounts of time to resolve, it is then described as chronic. This does not mean that progress will not be made with adequate treatment.

Among the drugs used for difficult-to-treat disease are doxycycline and tetracycline given in higher doses, or the macrolides, such as clarithromycin (the generic form of Biaxin) or azithromycin, both given in combination with the antimalarial drug hydroxychloroquine (the generic form of Plaquenil), which has been shown to enhance penetration of macrolides into cells.

Untreated Lyme disease can be transmitted during pregnancy, as documented by the Lyme disease pediatrician Charles Ray Jones, and confirmed by the experience of many families. Although the Infectious Diseases Society of America says there is no evidence for gestational Lyme, families with Lyme-infected infants and children strongly disagree. Pregnant women with Lyme disease, or exposed to Lyme disease, need to be treatedwith an antibiotic that is safe to use during pregnancy. This is true for breast-feeding women as well.

From the outset, I made it clear that I wanted aggressive treatment. I had no illusions that my disease would be cured easily. It did not respond to low doses, and I had gone into the disease healthy and with no allergies. When I was on an intravenous antibiotic and progress was slow, I sometimes had an oral antibiotic as well, ciprofloxacin, for example, for wider-spectrum coverage. When I was on intravenous vancomycin, I had an accompanying drug in the penicillin family. There was no way to know what strains of the Borrelia I had, or the degree of virulence of the bacteria in my body. My disease was difficult to treat and the benefits of higher doses were very evident.

Other oral drugs are also used for treating Lyme disease, and amounts that are given may need to be increased. Individual experiences with this disease differ widely. Some of the oral antibiotics that I used were Biaxin with Plaquenil, and tetracycline, changing at intervals according to my response. I also used Zithromax. Sometimes I changed from tetracycline to Biaxin because of stomach irritation, or for my doctor to assess whether a change would increase the rate of progress. For improvement, I required high levels of antibiotics on a continuing basis. I saw what happened to some who stopped, or interrupted, their treatment, or cut their pills in half, and I was unwilling to take unnecessary chances.

Intravenous drugs are also given for treating the disease. Rocephin, the trade name for ceftriaxone, is the one most frequently used. Brian Fallon found that 10 weeks of Rocephin resulted in statistical improvement in Spect scans. The IDSA recognizes its possible need, and it's the one it recommends, but only for a duration of days or weeks, not months. With entrenched disease, a short course of antibiotics, intravenous or oral, cannot be expected to be effective. Other intravenous antibiotics can be used as well, as described in the ILADS treatment guidelines.

The Lyme Disease Association and the International Lyme and Associated Diseases Society are sources of treatment guides for persistent or chronic Lyme disease. Physicians who treat it have wide clinical experience with the antibiotics used for Lyme disease, and many have researched their effectiveness. However, federal funding for long-term, controlled treatment studies is needed, and most of the research proposals have been denied except for the flawed and frequently challenged studies done by physicians who are associated with the Infectious Diseases Society of America.

As always, treatment decisions must be made in close partnership with the physician, both doing the best job they can. I knew that I was getting the best treatment available for my condition, and that my disease had been made far worse because of my experience with the IDSA guidelines that had left me ill and undiagnosed with no more than four weeks of doxycycline.

There is no easy answer for treatment for all Lyme disease. There can be no one protocol that fits all, and we don't yet have the research we need. Lyme patients are required to use the clinical experience and the research results that we have. It may not be all that we would want, but my treatment was based on the experience of thousands of patients with chronic Lyme, along with my responses to it.

THE JARISCH-HERXHEIMER REACTION TO ANTIBIOTICS

Progress can sometimes be hard to determine, especially with late disease, and patience is often required. The complex nature of the spirochete, including its many forms and surface proteins, allows it to survive while sequestered from antibiotics for long periods of time in which patients may remain symptom free. Its reproduction time is from twelve to twenty-four hours, making it less accessible to antibiotics than other bacteria (in contrast, streptococcus and staphylococcus bacteria divide every twenty minutes). Most antibiotics inhibit formation of cell walls and are therefore effective only when the bacteria divide, forming a new cell membrane. Therefore, if they divide only infrequently, they are less susceptible to the antibiotic than are bacteria that divide often.

The Jarisch-Herxheimer reaction is thought to be due to the response of the spirochete to the antibiotic. As bacteria are killed, they produce a toxin that has been found similar to that of botulism, with the result that Lyme flares can be intense. This response was first noted with syphilis spirochetes. When an antibiotic is given, symptoms may at first increase. With Lyme disease, the "herx" response (abbreviation for the Jarisch-Herxheimer reaction) can be strong enough to derail treatment either temporarily or permanently, for patients who don't know about it.

Patients may not accept even two weeks of treatment if they feel worse after taking the medicine. The decision may be made, mistakenly, to cut back or eliminate treatment, seeking answers instead from rheumatologists, gastroenterologists, and others. Visits to these specialists to address Lyme symptoms rarely result in diagnosis and therefore no antibiotics are given.

The reaction may occur at any time during treatment, and be brief or long-lasting. The erroneous conclusion can be that the antibiotic is not working, that it is making the patient sick, or that the patient is allergic to the antibiotic. On the other hand, especially in early disease, symptoms may improve quickly after starting antibiotics, and there will be no "herx" reaction. The good news, though, is that it helps confirm diagnosis of the disease. Much about it remains unknown, though no one doubts that it exists, but as with other aspects of Lyme disease, funding goes in other directions.

MY EXPERIENCE WITH THE
JARISCH-HERXHEIMER REACTION

When I was diagnosed and started antibiotics, I was forewarned that I might get worse before I got better. I was told that symptoms that I had earlier, and could have forgotten, might return. Bob, the counselor at a New Jersey home care service, where at any one time as many as a hundred Lyme patients were on intravenous antibiotics, some in wheelchairs, gave me much-needed support. Tirelessly, Bob returned my phone calls, told me about Lyme disease in his family, and reassured me that the antibiotic was doing its job if either I got better or I got worse. If my symptoms didn't change, the news was less good. He urged me to "hang in."

Within a week or two of starting treatment, my knees swelled, first one knee and then the other. My headaches also increased. Several months later, when I began eight months of intravenous treatment, the reaction was so strong that I went to the hospital for pain relief. The pain medications that I was offered, however, were those that I had already tried and found useless. They had been ordered by doctors I had seen earlier, but who had not diagnosed my disease. As I recall, one was Naprosyn, a drug used for mild or moderate pain for such conditions as rheumatoid arthritis or osteoarthritis. The other was Seldane, not a pain medication but an antihistamine that the Food and Drug Administration withdrew from the market in 1997 because of possible cardiac events, especially if used with the antibiotic erythromycin.

For me, as with many others with Lyme disease, pain medications offered little or no relief. When I went to the hospital I had been taking tetracycline for four months. I had just changed to the intravenous antibiotic Rocephin (ceftriaxone) and had been on it for about three weeks. My legs burned as though they were pressed against a hot iron, and my knees felt as though nails were being pounded into my kneecaps. At the emergency room I told them I had Lyme disease and had such pain that something needed to be done for relief. I don't know what the admitting doctor thought, but he recorded my information.

While at the hospital, I had medical tests, including an MRI, which is harder to obtain on an outpatient basis and requires waiting for scheduled appointments. It showed nothing wrong, and all my blood tests continued to be normal, as they always had been. The hospital staff appeared to accept my Lyme disease diagnosis. At least, there was no argument. I explained the intravenous procedure that I was following to the hospital's intravenous nurse. I had brought saline flushes with me in case they didn't have them available at the hospital. I didn't want to take the chance of my line getting blocked and had been instructed by the nurse at the home care company to use the flushes regularly. But on the third day, without explanation to me or contact with my Lyme disease physician, the daily antibiotic did not appear. The conversation went like this:

"Where is my Rocephin?"
"Dr. Smithline [the admitting physician] has taken you off it."
"I need to have it."
"You'll have to talk to him."
"When will he come back?"
"Tomorrow."
"I want to leave the hospital."
"If you leave the hospital against medical advice, your insurance won't pay for your hospital stay."

Although experienced in advocating for patient rights, I was put to the test with Lyme disease. For years, I had educated parents and hospitals for better maternity care, taught preparation for childbirth classes, provided hospital labor support, enabled access to babies through rooming-in programs, and written books providing information to the public on how to get the care they wanted as well as explaining to doctors and hospitals the need for change.

But now I was in a world I could not have dreamed of when I discovered the tick the preceding May. This was January, eight months after discovering the attached tick. My clothes were in a locker. I had no money or keys. I called a friend to pick me up at the hospital entrance. I didn't know whether the nurses were bluffing or not about the insurance company not paying, and didn't take the time to find out. I planned to return to the hospital, and if there was a problem I would deal with it later and do whatever was necessary. If I could not return, I already knew the hospital had nothing to offer me. The threat did not affect my decision and may have even strengthened my determination. The doctor had not even talked to me before withdrawing my medicine. Putting my coat over my hospital gown, I moved quickly out of the unit into an elevator to the first floor and out to the waiting car. My friend in the car asked, "Is this legal?"

While I was making arrangements to leave, my hospital roommate, receiving intravenous chemotherapy, listened with interest to my telephone calls but said nothing. If nurses came looking for me, I knew she would tell them. I didn't dare take the time to get dressed. I hoped the car would be there, and it was, with engine running. I opened the door and slid in quickly, settling back with a sigh of relief. Arriving home in less than twenty minutes on that snowy January morning I took my intravenous antibiotic and returned to the hospital, arriving an hour-and-a-half later. Two security people stood at the door. I walked past them into the elevator and up to my unit where two nurses were standing at the door of my unit. I had a bag with me that contained saline flushes and a note book with telephone numbers. Without saying anything, the nurses took the bag from me and emptied it on the counter of the nurses' station. They kept the flushes and note book without comment but returned the bag.

Dr. Smithline arrived within minutes. He sat in the chair by the bed. I said only that I had to take care of my Lyme disease. He didn't say much of anything and didn't mention his order to withdraw the order for the medicine. I didn't say anything more but started eating lunch that was on a tray by the bed, staying calm and trying to keep my hand from shaking. I didn't know what was going to happen. He sat silently for a few minutes and then left. I could only assume that he did not accept the Lyme disease diagnosis, or the need for treatment, thinking the antibiotic was making me sick. I was discharged from the hospital the following day, and continued Rocephin treatment as planned. Months later, my husband saw Dr. Smithline again. He asked only, "How is her arthritis?"

KEEPING IN MIND THE IDSA POSITION

The IDSA guidelines contain a certain amount of what appears as double talk, making them confusing for clinicians. For example, they mention longer-term antibiotics (meaning weeks, not months) but then recommend against them, speaking of the harm that may occur, as with an allergic reaction to amoxicillin (such as hives, difficulty breathing). They say there is no evidence of congenital Lyme disease. Many families with sick children would disagree. Their children were born with Lyme disease.

The guidelines speak of requiring spinal taps and testing of synovial fluid in the knee, even though spirochetes are hardly ever found in spinal or synovial fluid, even with polymerase chain reaction testing for DNA. As is generally the case, mine was negative, even with my raging symptoms of weakness, dizziness, knee joint pain, swollen knees, headache, and sweats. They do not diagnose Lyme disease, and evidence indicates strongly that in late Lyme disease the spirochetes are most likely sequestered inside cells, especially nerve cells.

Even with serious disease, their guidelines are restrictive. For example, "Adult patients with late neurological [Lyme] disease affecting the central or peripheral nervous system should be treated with ceftriaxone (2 g once per day intravenously for 2–4 weeks) ... Response to treatment is usually slow and may be incomplete. Re-treatment is not recommended unless relapse is shown by reliable objective measures." No definition is given for "reliable objective measures."

Considering how very sick some people are, requiring months and longer of intravenous therapy for improvement, and even longer for cure, this arbitrary limitation to two weeks appears almost ludicrous. How can one even consider simply stopping treatment for late neurological Lyme disease in two weeks?

Regarding cardiac symptoms, the same rule applies. "Patients with atrioventricular heart block may be treated with either oral or parenteral [intravenous] antibiotic therapy for 14 days (range 14–21 days)." Hospitalization and monitoring are recommended. "For advanced heart block [due to Lyme] a temporary pacemaker may be required; expert consultation with a cardiologist is recommended." As with late neurological Lyme disease, those with heart block, if following IDSA guidelines, would be limited to three weeks of treatment and asked to accept a "temporary" pacemaker. For those who treat serious Lyme and for those who have experience Lyme disease-caused heart block, this recommendation is unacceptable.

The IDSA says "Lyme arthritis" that continues after twenty-eight days of oral antibiotic should be re-treated with another four-week course of oral antibiotics or with a two- to four-week intravenous antibiotic, followed by a second four-week course for those who show improvement. "Clinicians should consider waiting several months before initiating retreatment with antimicrobial agents because of the anticipated slow resolution of inflammation after treatment." With this view of the illness, insurance companies benefit because less treatment is given and delay is recommended before re-treatment, but patients undergo other medical costs for untreated disease that are far greater than those of oral antibiotics and, patients cannot expect to recover from Lyme disease as they would if treatment was not interrupted or stopped.

The startling IDSA conclusion is that "to date, there is no convincing biologic evidence for the existence of chronic B. burgdorferi infection among patients after receipt of recommended treatment regimens for Lyme disease." The presence of Lyme spirochetes in the form of cysts is not acknowledged, nor is the research demonstrating the persistence of infection. No acknowledgment is made of the difficulty in finding spirochetes in blood or body tissues.

SUCCESS RATES

Symptoms vary and may recur. Many are subjective and can't be measured by laboratory tests or X-rays. No laboratory can tell you when the infection is gone. Those on the other side of the controversy say about recovered patients, "You can't prove whether people ever had Lyme disease, so the fact that they are now well is meaningless. They probably didn't have Lyme in the first place." They can say that because of the testing problem. We don't have the reliable ones that we need.

There is no way to tell by a test whether or not the patient is still infected. If the patient has a positive Western blot after being treated, those on the other side can say, and they do, "Just because he has a positive Western Blot does not mean that he still has active infection." Fortunately, people do recover from Lyme, even with long-undiagnosed and undertreated disease. In Boston University's publication, *Bostonia,* Sam Donta says, "It takes eighteen months of treatment on average to cure the disease." The article continues, regarding Donta's two practices, "Donta has prescribed lengthy course of antibiotics for patients for fifteen years. About 75 per cent of the patients he treats show improvement, and a quarter are symptom-free."[2] Donta found similar results in his 2005 study of a hundred patients at Falmouth (Massachusetts) Hospital.

Donta has studied both tetracycline therapy and macrolide therapy for Lyme disease. About the macrolides, his study results say, "80 percent of patients had self-reported improvement of 50 percent or more at the end of three months." As I previously stated, macrolides are used in combination with an antimalarial drug to raise intracellular pH (to make it more alkaline). When macrolides or hydroxychloroquine were used alone, there was no improvement.[3] In his study of 277 patients on tetracycline, he found that a "history of longer duration of symptoms or antibiotic treatment was associated with longer treatment times to achieve improvement and cure.[4] After two months, 33 percent of patients' conditions were significantly improved. After three months, 61 percent of the patients' conditions were significantly improved.

Lesley Fein's study, "Retrospective Analysis of 160 Patients with Lyme Disease," is a treatment study in which extensive laboratory and clinical data were collected at the initial visit and at three month intervals for one year during and after treatment. A variety of antibiotics were used in this study: Biaxin, Zithromax, Amoxicillin, Claforan, Rocephin, Vancomycin, intramuscular bicillin LA, Plaquenil, Suprax, and Ceftin. A favorable patient response was directly proportional to the length of treatment. At the time of initial diagnosis, only 70 percent of patients were seropositive. During therapy, the ultimate seropositive rate became 99.4 percent.

Data support the clinical observation; Lyme disease is diagnosed on the basis of clinical criteria. A significant number present as seronegative and only seroconvert months into therapy, often when in remission. Treatment must be tailored to the individual patient. An improved response with therapy of longer duration and repeated courses of treatment is clearly documented by this study.

Charles Ray Jones, who has treated over six thousand children with Lyme, says that three quarters are well after three months to seven years of treatment, averaging nine months to two years. The remaining quarter is still receiving treatment, most of whom have been denied health insurance coverage.

The *Lyme Times* reported back in 1998 that "Dr. Burrascano [who began treating Lyme in the mid-1980s] has studied the effect of lengthened duration of treatment and established a direct relationship between duration and success, starting at 17 percent for one month of therapy and reaching a plateau at 67 percent at five months of duration."[5] His figures are currently being updated.

In 2004, The International Lyme and Associated Diseases Society published evidence-based guidelines for Lyme disease, a handbook for physicians and medical care providers. It says, "Because of the dis-appointing long-term outcome with shorter courses of antibiotics, the practice of stopping antibiotics to allow for a delayed recovery is no longer recommended for patients with persistent, recurrent, and refractory Lyme disease. Reports show failure rates of 30–62 percent within three years of short-course treatment using antibiotics thought to be effective for Lyme disease."

About the severity of chronic Lyme disease, the ILADS guidelines say,

> For patients with chronic Lyme disease, the quality of life has been evaluated in a clinical trial sponsored by the National Institutes of Health using a standardized questionnaire. The so-designated quality of life of the 107 individuals with chronic Lyme disease was worse than that of patients with type 2 diabetes or a recent heart attack, and equivalent to that of patients with congestive heart failure or osteoarthritis.

With correct information in hand, the public cannot accept the common responses to a tick bite and rash, with all the potential associated risks: "This can't be Lyme. You don't need more treatment. You've had enough. You probably have some arthritis. It may be a muscle strain. Come back if it doesn't go away."

Because the other side claims to have settled the issue, promulgated their own guidelines that are favored by the insurance companies, and concluded that there is no chronic Lyme disease, those requiring long-term care continue to face the overwhelming problem of trying to find a doctor and explaining the controversy to almost everyone.

The next chapter tells you some of my experiences in coping with long-term disease, including taking antibiotics intravenously, diet and exercise, and physical therapy. I discuss insurance coverage and provide testimony from the insurance industry on its use of the IDSA guidelines.

CHAPTER NINE

LIVING WITH PERSISTENT LYME DISEASE

INSURANCE AND LIFESTYLE ISSUES

Irwin Vanderhoof, PhD, Professor at the New York University Stern School of Business, estimates that Lyme disease costs society about $1 billion per year. This includes unnecessary or inappropriate medical care, lost productivity, legal fees, and other direct / indirect expenses. However, the human toll can be high. Patients can have ongoing problems, resulting in emotional distress, permanent physical damage, and significant disruption of life (e.g., job loss, divorce, loss of friends, or family).

—IRWIN VANDERHOOF, _CONTINGENCIES_[1]

Contingencies is an actuarial trade publication for the insurance industry. The study was done by the Lyme Disease Foundation. The LDF worked on the study for two years and results were confirmed by subsequent studies.

Since 1993, the estimates of costs to society have doubled, and are currently about $2 billion a year, including diagnosis, treatment, and lost wages.

By not acknowledging chronic Lyme, however, we can't know the true price. As I have discussed, conservatively, at least 10 percent and more of cases become chronic. In addition, many are unaware that re-ported cases represent only new ones and do not include those who develop chronic disease and continue to be sick.

If the disease progresses, life becomes more difficult. Ted says, "I went to a family reunion and was so exhausted that I spent most of the time upstairs in bed." Lisa says, "I tried to type a power of attorney, but everything became blurry, and I made typos on every line." Getting un-derstanding from others is not always possible, especially over a long pe-riod of time, and with no visible symptoms, such as a broken leg. People can't add. They can't remember. They have ringing in the ears, tremors and vertigo, all the while seeking disability payments for a disease that is barely acknowledged.

The very diagnosis may be challenged and the treatment stopped. The fact that many don't respond promptly to treatment casts doubts in the minds of some that the disease can even be Lyme. For example, in January 2002, I attended a Boston Hospital lecture at which Allen Steere, the pioneer in Lyme disease, presented a case of a fifty-nine-year-old man who had been a financial planner before he contracted Lyme disease. He was given tetracycline for seven weeks, relapsed, and was re-treated. The antibiotic was then stopped, despite a long list of continuing neurological symptoms. Instead the man was treated psychologically with "cognitive restructuring," a process used for those with such conditions as depression, trauma, and social phobias to redi-rect the thinking process. Steere then discussed stress management and lifestyle change. That morning several dozen medical professionals were given the message, although unstated, that the patient no longer has Lyme. The patient is disabled, but the cause is denied.

NEWSWEEK ADDRESSES "THE GREAT LYME DEBATE"

In August 2007, Newsweek reported on the controversy that prevents many from receiving medical treatment for ongoing Lyme disease. In the article, Gary Wormser, who chaired the IDSA panel on its restric-tive guidelines, speaks on the issues. "There's no such thing as chronic

Lyme, because in most patients who complain of it, Borrelia isn't detectable in the body." (This is true. Spirochetes can hardly ever be found in those with Lyme disease.) "The majority of patients treated for 'chronic Lyme' do not have post-Lyme," he says, "and in fact, never, ever had Lyme disease at all." Wormser concludes by saying, "The guidelines represent the best that medical science has to offer."

The *Newsweek* article continued, "Raphael Stricker, however, president of the International Lyme and Associated Diseases Society, believes in 'chronic Lyme disease' and says that in his clinical experience about 70 percent of patients treated get better if they're treated long term with the same drugs used to treat early infection."

In the same article, *Newsweek* further says,

> Richard Blumenthal, attorney general of Connecticut, has launched an investigation of the IDSA panel, looking into whether it ignored research that would support long-term antibiotic treatment. "Our question basically is whether the guidelines were formulated through a process that was proper, without self-interest or conflicts of interest," Blumenthal says, noting that some of the panel members have financial interests in treatments and vaccines. He also worries that the guidelines might be used by insurance companies looking to avoid paying for Lyme drugs.[2]

YOUR FIRST RESPONSIBILITY

Antibiotics are the only recognized means of cure. I had directions for taking mine, and I didn't deviate or forget. I obtained refills well before the bottle was empty and didn't take "days off" to "give my body a rest." At times, those with Lyme fear that they are taking "too many antibiotics" and interrupt treatment unnecessarily, deciding to let their immune systems handle the disease. With the exception of treatment regimens that include this plan, or Jarisch-Herxheimer reactions that become too strong, there is no benefit in taking "days off," any more than there is for those being treated for tuberculosis. The focus cannot be on "feeling better" because that can take a very long time. Some leave treatment because they no longer have insurance. "If I can get a job with medical benefits, I'll go back on treatment."

LIFESTYLE AND HEALTH ISSUES

Having Lyme disease does not mean that medical care for other conditions stops. It is sometimes difficult to know what is Lyme and what isn't, but, whenever possible, routine medical visits and tests should continue. Whatever is happening with Lyme disease, the need for rest, exercise, and healthy foods does not go away.

Lyme disease typically causes fatigue, and often insomnia as well, where sleeping for any length of time can be nearly impossible. With late hours, and stress-inducing commitments, many report their Lyme symptoms become worse. Recovery from increased responsibilities may require a couple of days or more. Setting priorities and simplifying life helps control the stress inherent in having this disease.

Despite pain and fatigue, the known benefits of exercise, including improved blood circulation, require that those with Lyme attempt to move, walk, and do whatever they can. Muscle weakness is a symptom of the disease, and with persistent Lyme, muscle tone may be diminished despite efforts to maintain former strength. Exercise usually results in an improved feeling of well-being. Too much, however, can result in fatigue and pain. The individual must judge.

SOME OF MY EXPERIENCES IN COPING WITH LYME

After months mostly spent in bed, I decided to go to an orthopedist to have my knees X-rayed again, not that the results, whatever they were, would change anything. The elevator to the fourth floor office wasn't working so I struggled up four flights of stairs. The X-rays were normal and the physician was puzzled at the evident knee swelling.

When I said it was because of Lyme, he looked doubtful. He said he had never seen a case of Lyme disease and suggested that the physical therapist could give me electrical therapy. He didn't know how it worked, but it was something the physical therapists did. I made an appointment. Although it is important to rule out causes of symptoms that could be something other than Lyme, I found it frustrating once again to realize that the specialists that I visited didn't recognize my illness and saw me as having no problem.

I lay on my back while the therapist drew my legs up at right angles, one at a time, hurting every inflamed nerve in my legs. I couldn't ride the bicycle at all and failed every balance test miserably. My knees were wrapped, and an electrical current was introduced causing a feeling of "pins and needles." I went for three sessions with no apparent results. The physical therapist was kind but puzzled. Like the orthopedist, she knew nothing of Lyme.

Despite pain, physical exercise, even though minimal, is necessary to maintain health, strength, and blood circulation. When I could, I resumed my membership at the health club and used the swimming pool daily, including the hot tub and sauna. Lyme spirochetes do not like heat, as with high body temperature. Although there's no way of knowing whether saunas help those with Lyme disease, they did, however, increase my comfort level. I dealt with pain by using hot water bottles that I found far more effective than heating pads.

As time passed, I became able to use some of the weight-training machines, which I had used before my illness. Later, I found that I could ride a horse in the ring, or go on a short trail ride, but practicalities such as transportation and possible safety risks along with lack of stamina prevented me from continuing this activity. With easier access, it would have been an ideal activity for me to pursue on a regular basis for balance, back strengthening, and relaxation.

FOOD AND NUTRITION

Some antibiotics are taken with food and cannot be taken on an empty stomach, for example, doxycycline and Biaxin. Others, such as tetracycline, require an empty stomach, and as described previously, are not taken with milk- and calcium-containing medications. It is important that you get good instructions from your doctor. I had to keep reminding myself as I balanced food requirements with my medication schedule, especially when I was taking more than one antibiotic at a time. For a while I was taking Biaxin along with supplementary vitamin C, until I learned that the drug requires a high intracellular pH to be most effective, and must not be taken with citrus fruit or vitamin C. Information comes from physicians, and pharmacists are excellent resources as well.

Lyme may affect appetite and alter food choices. At times the disease may cause nausea. Sometimes antibiotics can, too. I always continued to eat whether or not I was hungry, and if I went too long without food, my stomach could become uncomfortable. I kept a generous supply of a variety of high-quality foods that were easy to prepare, eating whatever appealed to me. I had whole grain breads and cereals, milk, yogurt, cheese, tuna, juices, hard-boiled eggs, fruit, vegetables, and soups. I did not try to cook evening meals, and, if I was alone, take-out meals were available that could be delivered. I took great care to have high-quality food in my house and eat a balanced diet. Antibiotics are essential, but maintaining a healthy lifestyle is critical as well.

GOING THE INTRAVENOUS ROUTE

I had no doubt that the corkscrew bacteria had gone far beyond my bloodstream, and I had no expectation that I would be well in four weeks. After a month I no longer experienced a pounding, racing heart, and after four months my general body strength was better, and I wasn't dizzy or light-headed, but pain was intense. I started on an intravenous antibiotic. They have not been found necessarily more effective than oral medications, but may be used as a result of delayed diagnosis because they are delivered directly into the body.

At first, giving my own IV was daunting, especially when I was almost too sick to read the manual. People who need daily infusions over a period of time, for any medical reason, do them at home, and I was acquainted with those who had done this for other reasons. The intravenous nurse from the home care company taught me the procedure, and I had a twenty-four-hour telephone number to call if I needed answers, or a nurse to come to my home. Every week a van appeared in my driveway to deliver medical supplies in a white foam box lined with cold packs.

The home care nurse also came weekly, sometimes trudging through snow, to check me and change the dressing. She said that I was not the first Lyme patient that she had visited, but that most of her patients had lines in place for other conditions, such as those unable to take food by mouth, or persisting infections that were not caused by Lyme. A thin, flexible catheter was inserted into a vein in my forearm and threaded up the vein to my shoulder. It remained in place for me to attach the bag of medicine each day. Instructions included hand washing with antibacterial soap, drying with paper towels, and using alcohol wipes and saline flushes. When I was finished with my infusion each morning, I detached the empty bag of antibiotic and threw it away. Left in place was the device to which I attached the line, with a dressing at the site where the line entered my arm. I wore an arm band that concealed it. Wearing long sleeves makes the infusion site invisible to others. I took tub baths with my arm hanging over the edge to keep it dry. Some people take showers with a plastic sleeve over the dressing. If the dressing loosens for any reason, such as from perspiration on a hot day, or because Lyme disease may cause sweats, the nurse comes to replace it.

Travel out of town may be done, with the line in place, by bringing along supplies and medicine, finding a refrigerator at your destination, and chilling the medicine with cold packs. Patients have come to Lyme disease conferences with their catheters and medicines.

After I'd been on a daily intravenous antibiotic for about three months, a friendly and cheerful woman from the insurance company called to ask, "Are you still getting daily IVs?" "Yes." "How long do you think you'll be doing this?" I had to guess. I said I had chronic Lyme disease. "Maybe three more months." My answer brought an immediate "Okay." Actually, I had to be on intravenous antibiotics far longer, but my insurance company always paid every medical charge. I was not required to provide documentation, have my doctor write letters of medical necessity, or go through the lengthy appeal process that is required when claims are denied.

I had private health insurance and was not in a managed care plan. When I signed up for the intravenous treatment, the financial person at the home care company made arrangements with my insurance company, and I was not involved in the process. The company approved it without an end or limit, but managed care plans are likely to be less cooperative.

The cost of intravenous therapy averages several thousand dollars per week. Home care is a labor-intensive process. I have never seen the breakdown, but home care nurses cover wide geographic areas. My nurse sometimes traveled twenty miles between patients, along with bringing equipment into each home for dressing changes and taking temperatures and blood pressures. In addition each week a delivery person also came with a refrigerated box containing bags of antibiotic solution and other supplies involved in the daily infusion. Some have paid expenses out of pocket to continue their treatment. Compared to costs of heart surgery, brain surgery, and cancer, for which there are few insurance claim problems, the high costs for intravenous Lyme disease therapy must be kept in perspective with expensive therapy that is allowed without question for other serious conditions.

"I was doing well on intravenous treatment, but they pulled my line after a month." Since that time, this man's insurance company has paid for endocrine studies, gastrointestinal CAT scans, neurological studies, and brain scans, along with ongoing physician visits. These added expenses may have been unnecessary had the therapy been completed. And if he had been diagnosed earlier before his disease became chronic, there would have been no expectation that he would require intravenous treatment.

THE INSURANCE INDUSTRY AND LYME DISEASE

The November 27, 2004, hearing on chronic Lyme disease, conducted by the New York State Assembly on Health, and chaired by Richard Gottfried, included testimony by Kenneth Liegner, Robert Bransfield, Brian Fallon, and Steven Phillips. No Infectious Diseases Society of America physicians testified. The New York State Health Department did not send a representative, saying, "We don't really have anything to say on this topic; we just follow CDC guidelines."

At the hearing, for the first time, a representative from the insurance industry, Dr. Alan Muney, spoke publicly. His testimony left no doubt why those who have Lyme disease risk being left with uncertain insurance coverage, despite legislation that has been passed in Rhode Island and Connecticut, which addresses long-term treatment for Lyme disease. He spoke on behalf of Oxford Health Plans, espousing the IDSA's position on limiting treatment for Lyme disease. He laid out his case in fifty-five pages of testimony, using the word *evidence* thirty-four times, the word *guidelines* twenty-three times, and the words *expert* or *expert testimony* many more times. Legislators persisted in asking him, "What evidence?" "Whose guidelines?" and "Whose experts?"

Muney explained the insurance industry's position that denies or limits payment for Lyme disease, admitting to a very large epidemic and that these were just the reported cases. He admitted to unknowns in Lyme disease, and that symptoms may persist after treatment. He knew what the treatment should be, if in fact the patient really did have Lyme "because the insurance industry follows guidelines."

Oxford Health Plans, his company, he said received 500 requests for intravenous antibiotics for late-stage Lyme disease. Seventy-three percent were approved, and of the fifty-seven cases denied, fifty were upheld when referred to external review. When asked what the treatment was for the 73 percent approved cases, he said that those approved might get six weeks, although this is beyond the guidelines. Oxford would "approve antibiotic treatment intravenously, that is up to six weeks treatment—actually both oral and intravenous treatment combined."

The following dialogue occurred between Dr. Muney and members of the New York State Assembly on Health at the November 27, 2001, hearing on chronic Lyme disease in Albany. Members of the committee were fully cognizant of the chronic Lyme disease problem in their state, and they questioned Dr. Muney extensively about his position on providing medical insurance coverage for Lyme disease. Chairman Richard Gottfried and Joel Miller of the committee presided over another hearing in Manhattan two months later on January 31, 2002, New York's Office of Professional Medical Conduct's process on investigation of mainstream doctors that had resulted in prosecution of the Lyme physician Joseph Burrascano.

> ASSEMBLYMAN GOTTFRIED: But the company's policy would be that if there was a request from a patient, based on a treatment recommendation by the patient's board certified rheumatologist, what have you, for longer treatment than the initial six weeks, Oxford's policy would be to deny that and to provide it only if your judgment were—the company's judgment were overturned by internal review or external review?

> DR. MUNEY: That is correct because the current practice guidelines—again, the ones put out, as I said, by the Infectious Diseases Society of America, the CDC, the American College of Physicians—all state that. So—

> GOTTFRIED: These guidelines state that longer than six weeks is never appropriate?

MUNEY: The current guidelines that are in place will say, for example, for late Lyme disease, there's—you get a month's worth of oral therapy or a month's worth of parenteral [intravenous] therapy. If you have a reoccurrence [sic] you actually can get more therapy, another month of either as well. So these are the guidelines that are in place.

GOTTFRIED: How many patients that remained ill would it take to convince the insurance companies that there might be a problem? Is it ten patients, is it 100 patients, or is [sic] the 10,000 patients in New York State alone that seem to continue to have these problems?

ASSEMBLYMAN JOEL MILLER: So, if you have someone—and we need to hear that, you know, twenty-eight days of antibiotic and you're cured; right? I mean we had [Raymond] Dattwyler out at Stonybrook said [sic] 28 days of treatment and now you're cured, and you have no additional invasion by a microorganism and then suddenly you begin to show symptoms again? So you haven't been reinfected, but now you're not cured. So, there we had an expert opinion. It happened to be what was widely believed at one point not long ago. And now the person is showing symptoms again—not new infection, the same old infection. Obviously this wasn't cured. And this can go on and on. How do you determine the exact length of time when someone is cured based on evidence-based evidence you like, from the experts you like, if, in fact, they keep getting sick [with possible relapse]?

Assemblywoman Nettie Mayerson then spoke of physicians who take a position for continuing treatment because they believe they are helping their patients. Their position is based on hard medical experience, good physician practicing medicine.

The dialogue continued.

ASSEMBLYMAN [MICHAEL] COHEN: Dr. [Kenneth] Liegner [in earlier testimony] referred to a seven-year old patient that [*sic*] was receiving intravenous antibiotics for a
period of, I believe, six months, and there was a physician
reviewer for the corporation, which denied further intravenous treatment. And Dr. Liegner wrote a letter to this
physician—and if I could just read a few sentences.

"Mr. and Mrs. X, meaning the parents of the seven year
old child, cannot afford to pay for X's treatment unless
they are reimbursed by their insurance coverage. To sus-
pend treatment when this child is showing progress in
terms of diminished seizure frequency, resumption of
ability to take sustenance by mouth, and ability to talk is
both cruel and lacking in compassion. But more than this,
it is my considered opinion that for a physician to fail to
treat this patient intensively at this point, or to prevent
such treatment by one's actions as a third-party review
physician would constitute medical negligence."

ASSEMBLYWOMAN MAYERSON: Can you tell me if it's
kind of—is the practice for insurance companies to refer
what they see as inappropriate medical care by Lyme doctors to the OPMC? We're trying to find out how many
complaints are patient-initiated and how many complaints have been initiated by the insurance companies or
HMO's or whatever.

DR. MUNEY: I can tell you just a little bit about the process.
If a patient . . . complained to us, we try to get as much of
the medical record [*sic*] and send it out for independent
reviewers to look at. And then, if in the opinion of inde-

pendent reviewers, and if in the opinion of independent reviewers they noted there is a significant—in their opinion—quality problem, we refer to our regional quality management committee, which are [*sic*] made up of practicing physicians, not Oxford physicians, who look at what the issues were. And then they can decide, that this physician should be sent a letter—outline—maybe they—everything from you need more continuing education to it's such a serious offense that we want to go ahead and terminate them from the network. That, of course, happens rarely. There's also a due process part legally that we do within the health plan if it comes to that. We will refer something to OPMC if we have terminated a doctor from the network.

Dr. Muney's testimony refers to all physicians, not only Lyme disease physicians who treat chronic Lyme disease.

ASSEMBLYMAN COHEN: You know, once again, the public's negative attitude toward medical insurance companies—some of it's shared by myself. There's the following thought process: that the decisions to deny services—many of them, if not all of them, I'm sorry, many of them are arbitrary, the logic being as follows: If you're reversed, you're going to pay for the service. And if a person is denied and does not file appeal, and perhaps if they did file an appeal, there would have been a reversal. Well, this is money being saved by the insurance company.

DR. MUNEY: Uh-huh.

Dr. Liegner, an internist who has treated chronic Lyme disease for more than fifteen years, said,

I think if the denial of chronic Lyme disease was able to—
[sic] were able to put an end to the denial of chronic Lyme,
I think we all could move forward and hopefully, people
could all work together to try to solve the very serious
problems that confront us.

And I would just like to say that I don't even think
that the enemy is the insurance industry, because I think
they are in a very tough spot. They really are in a tough
spot. I think we should have some sympathy for the insurance industry. They are faced with a massive epidemic
of very, very serious, life-threatening—and [sic] illness
that can either threaten life and can damage neurologi-
cally irreversibly. If they were—forced to confront their
responsibilities to their insured's, they actually could go
bankrupt.

About PCR (DNA) tests for Lyme, Dr. Liegner concluded by
saying,

. . . although PCR has been around in Lyme disease for at
least ten years, and it is widely used for many infectious
diseases without question, when it comes to Lyme disease
the PCR is suspect. And why is it suspect? Because the insurance companies—first of all they will not even reimburse a patient for getting a PCR, so that puts another
obstacle. And then once they get a PCR, their physician
consultants question the credibility of the laboratory,
even though the laboratories that we used participate in
and satisfy the College of American Pathology's profi-
ciency testing programs.

The single greatest obstacle to badly needed progress in
development of improved methods of diagnosis and

treatment for Lyme disease is the chronic persistent denial of chronic persistent infection in this illness.

The next chapter addresses the much-touted issue of "taking too many antibiotics." This is a genuine concern in our society, but does not apply to Lyme. Lyme disease does not become resistant to these medicines.

CHAPTER TEN

"WHAT ABOUT ANTIBIOTIC RESISTANCE?" "AREN'T ANTIBIOTICS DANGEROUS?"

ANTIBIOTICS USED FOR TREATING LYME DISEASE

After a tick bite and rash, I was treated for Lyme disease with doxycycline for four weeks. My doctor said that was more than enough, and I never got symptoms. But now, six months later, I have recurrent sore throats and sometimes blurred vision, and insomnia that I never had before. I don't dare take more antibiotics, and don't know that my doctor would even give them to me. I wouldn't know how to persuade him. Neither my eye doctor nor my primary care doctor see anything wrong with me.

—CALLER ON LYME INFORMATION TELEPHONE LINE

The above statement, or some version of it, is representative of those who believe they did not receive enough treatment after a tick bite and don't understand symptoms they now have. They fear taking too many antibiotics, and don't know what to do for the health issues they are now experiencing. They don't know whether or not they still have Lyme.

Lyme disease requires antibiotics, and recurrence indicates the need for re-treatment as well. Subsequent occurrences may be recognized long after the initial infection, and symptoms may also be different from the original ones. It is hypothesized that a traumatic event, surgery, or another illness, may reactivate a dormant infection that is often unrecognized for what it is, the reappearance of Lyme disease. Even a DNA test cannot prove Lyme's existence, because, as we know, spirochetes can rarely be detected in the body. However, symptoms that make no sense for any other condition give the warning.

In August, 2007, the White House announced that President George W. Bush had Lyme the preceding year. He experienced a red rash with a light center below his left knee. He was treated, although the amount of medication given was not disclosed. It was thought he contracted the disease as a result of riding his bicycle in the woods of Maryland, which is the location of Camp David, the presidential retreat, and an area that is endemic for Lyme.

In the same article, the *New York Times* reported that Bush had bouts of unsteadiness after a viral infection, and that he had recovered from a serious bout of otitis media, which is an ear infection. The *Times* reported a White House spokesman as saying, "The president goes for lengthy bike rides on narrow trails in the woods and does not have any problems with his balance." The spokesman "likened President Bush's episodes of imbalance to the feeling that can occur in someone who has just gotten off a boat."

The *Times* said,

> The doctors attributed the unsteadiness to mild vestibular neuronitis in the president's left ear. The serious otitis media was in the right ear and was first detected last Friday, but has since cleared up. The sinusitis involved the right maxillary sinus.
>
> The findings are consistent with viral illnesses that can be followed by periods of unsteadiness for several weeks,

said Dr. Michael G. Stewart, the chief of ear, nose and
throat medicine at New York-Presbyterian/Weill Cornell
hospital. Untreated Lyme disease (said Dr. Stewart) can
lead to nerve damage, often involving the eighth cranial
nerve, the same one affected by vestibular neuronitis. But
Mr. Bush's doctors said they did not believe the Lyme infection was linked to his vestibular neuronitis because the
skin lesion had not recurred.

The article continued, "The White House doctors evaluated Mr.
Bush for Menière's disease, another ailment of the inner ear that can
produce vertigo, hearing loss and ringing in the ears. But doctors ruled
out Menière's disease because Mr. Bush did not have some key signs
and symptoms, the White House official said without disclosing what
they were."[1]

Lyme sufferers have these, or similar, symptoms, and if re-treatment
is unsuccessful seek evaluation by a Lyme-literate physician. Every case
is not the same and may require individual attention for treatment decisions, and an antibiotic beyond the standard doxycycline.

The described symptoms do not mean that Bush has Lyme disease.
However, in the *Times* article it is discounted for the reason that the rash
did not recur. The experience of Lyme patients shows that the reappearance of the rash, however, is uncommon. While it occurs early or
late, and lasts a short or longer time, and with possible multiple rashes
appearing later, typically it does not recur. The rash is not a measure of
whether or not the disease is cured.

It is not surprising that misinformation about Lyme disease continues, even in the most prestigious medical facilities. Doctors are told
that it is a short-term disease that does not become chronic. Fear of
"too many antibiotics" makes it easier to ignore continuing symptoms;
instead the search for another cause and a different diagnosis goes on.

Many who are symptom free, and think they are cured, still have
spirochetes in their bodies that can cause later symptoms. Large num-

bers of people carry Lyme bacteria in their bodies without any apparent symptoms, allowing the Lyme disease problem to seem innocuous (and the epidemic to remain invisible).

TAKING ANTIBIOTICS

The common questions about antibiotics are whether they are dangerous, and if taking them might cause antibiotic resistance, that overuse might make them ineffective in the future. Those with Lyme disease and their families may decide, unnecessarily, to discontinue antibiotics far too soon. For other conditions, directions call for taking all the medicine prescribed, even if the medical condition improves, rather than risk incomplete treatment. But because Lyme may require long courses of antibiotics, and the public lacks information on the risks of stopping treatment prematurely, the fear of taking "too many antibiotics" may prevail.

The decision may be reinforced by news articles. A *Cape Cod Times* article in which Bela Matya, medical director of epidemiology for the Massachusetts State Department of Public Health, said, "If you're going to have Lyme disease, it's probably best to have the rash so you can get diagnosed and treated early." The article quotes those who have Lyme disease, "Long-term Lyme sufferers say the disease turns their lives inside out, creating havoc with their memory, mobility, and general ability to function."

The article continued, "While the LDA [Lyme Disease Association] maintains that some patients need long-term treatment with antibiotics for Lyme disease, Sugar [Dr. Alan Sugar, chief of infectious disease at the Cape Cod Hospital] said that even second-stage Lyme disease responds well to shorter treatment." The article quoted him as saying, "After three weeks of treatment you're cured."[2]

With this information published on Cape Cod with its high rate of Lyme disease, it is no surprise the public might question the wisdom of taking long-term antibiotics. If the disease appears cured, some people may stop taking the medicine. Or, if their Lyme doesn't respond promptly to antibiotics, or they experience Jarisch-Herxheimer responses that temporarily increase symptoms, they may put the pills aside, fearing the antibiotic more than they do the disease.

MEDICATIONS TAKEN BY THE PUBLIC

Large numbers of over-the-counter medications are available to treat the common cold; more than eight hundred are on the market. Two billion dollars are spent annually on cough and cold medicines alone, the use of which has not declined since 1981. Yet increasing evidence demonstrates that these medications are not effective and may sometimes be harmful, especially to children.

Long-term drugs are given for gastric reflux disease, arthritis, depression, high blood pressure, attention deficit disorder, childhood hyperactivity, bipolar disorder, pain, and other conditions, although it is known that they may have significant side effects. Some of these medicines are taken for life.

Development of new drugs appears to have slowed, as reported in the *Boston Globe*. The potential market for a new antibiotic is an estimated $200 million to $400 million a year. "Pfizer sold $9.3 billion dollars of Lipitor, an anticholesterol treatment that is its best selling drug." The reason given for development of "lifestyle" drugs is that (in contrast to antibiotics) "a chronic condition such as high cholesterol or depression requires a pill every day for the rest of the patient's life."[3] Pills that are used indefinitely are infinitely more profitable than an investment in developing new antibiotics that are, for the most part, used for a limited period of time.

Development of antibiotics has diminished for several reasons. Among them is that Lyme disease research in general does not focus on treating the disease, and, without funding, new antibiotics that could be useful for this disease will not be available. The process of developing a new drug requires many steps, with a process in place for drug trials and post-marketing surveillance. Some say there is a preference for developing narrow-spectrum rather than broad-spectrum drugs, and new-drug costs are high. Many pharmaceutical companies' resources are used to promote drugs that are already on the market. Lyme disease is not a priority, especially when much of the literature says the disease is easily cured in a few weeks.

MEDICINE AND EVIDENCE

At the Albany hearing on chronic Lyme disease, Dr. Robert Bransfield, a psychiatrist specializing in working with treatment-resistant Lyme patients, said about medicine and evidence,

> What is called evidence-based medicine by the insurance industry today is not truly evidence-based medicine. Now, one argument I heard earlier was that you need double-blind studies to prove something. The reality is, most of medicine is not proven by double-blind studies. I'll give an example. Millions of people are treated with antidepressants to reduce risk of suicide. There has never been a single article, double-blind controlled study that proves that antidepressants reduce the risk of suicide. Now, if we went out and did a study like that it would be unethical. Once something is accepted, it's unethical to prove it by double-blind studies. So, we're in a quandary here. Most of medicine that's obvious, self-evident, does not fall into this category of double-blind research-proven. And when we're at the leading edge of medicine, we don't have double-blind studies supporting things. We didn't have a double-blind study that supported using the mechanical heart . . . would that have been a good idea? How can you ever do that? No, whenever we deal with people that are the difficult patients to treat, the challenging patients, we never have the luxury of evidence-based medicine. That comes long in the wake, when masses of people get involved after it's been established for many years. But we need to treat

people today, and we can't wait for evidence-based medicine to catch up with the realities of clinical practice.[4]

He addressed the placebo ("sugar pill") effect by saying, "as the study goes on over months, over a more extended time, then you see that dissipate. And when we're looking at Lyme, and we're looking at people that have this year after year, I think it's hard to discount everything as the placebo effect. I think that doesn't hold water."

OVERUSE OF ANTIBIOTICS

Of the antibiotics that are produced, 70 percent are mixed in animal feed with twenty-five million pounds used in feed for chickens, hogs, and beef cattle. The purpose is to promote somewhat faster growth in the animals, and compensate for crowded, unhealthy living conditions, conducive to spread of infections, of those that are raised on large-scale commercial farms. Humans ingest traces of these antibiotics in food, and antibiotics in animal feed can leach into groundwater, the source of our water supplies. These millions of pounds, used routinely, enter the food chain to put our planet at risk for the development of antibiotic-resistant bacteria. More than half of the antibiotics used in farming are important in treating human diseases, and overuse in animal feed contributes to antibiotic resistance to human infectious diseases. We are not using "too many antibiotics" for Lyme disease.

BACTERIAL RESISTANCE

Bacteria become resistant to antibiotics because strains of bacteria that are not killed survive and multiply. Surviving organisms may adapt in order to accommodate exposure to the drug. Continuing development of new antibiotics is required, and we need to preserve the ones that we have, making sure they are not used for viral (submicroscopic particles that cannot reproduce on their own) or other nonbacterial illnesses for which they are not effective. Practical considerations sometimes make this difficult. For example, a severe sore throat may, or may not, be due to a strep infection, but laboratory tests involve time and expense and do not meet the need for prompt treatment. Also, a bacterial infection may be present as well as a viral infection, and symptoms may become increasingly severe.

The difference between early and late Lyme disease treatment runs all the way from a rash and possible flulike symptoms to chronic disease and thousands of dollars for long-term treatment. The bacteria that are not eradicated early are less available to antibiotics after they have left the blood circulation. With this in mind, it makes sense to treat the disease aggressively.

Antibiotic resistance does not apply to Lyme as it does to many other infectious diseases because the disease is not spread person to person, except possibly during pregnancy. A person bitten by a tick becomes a "dead-end host" for the disease. Therefore, antibiotic-resistant strains cannot evolve. And because they do not evolve from treating Lyme disease, we do not have concerns about using them when they are needed. We are not using too many antibiotics. The common problem is delayed, inadequate, and incomplete treatment.

WHAT ABOUT SIDE EFFECTS?

Package inserts included with a multitude of drugs, and advertisements in the media for drugs, describe a variety of possible side effects. They leave no doubt that many commonly used drugs may result, for example, in heartburn, dizziness, nausea, stomach pain, change in bowel function, muscle weakness, insomnia, and others that are far more serious. They provide information on when to call your doctor, such as during high fever, choking, and loss of consciousness.

Antibiotics used for Lyme disease are no exception, but they are innocuous compared with many frequently used drugs, even when taken long term. Those who oppose extending treatment cite possible infections in the intravenous line, gall bladder problems, nausea, and diarrhea. Some antibiotics when used long term require routine periodic blood tests, such as checking liver enzyme levels.

They are substances that kill or injure bacteria using a variety of mechanisms such as interference with cell wall or DNA synthesis. Some have broad-spectrum action while others are more specific. More than a hundred are commonly used and fall into classes such as penicillins, tetracyclines, quinolones, sulfonamides, and others. Some work best on skin infections; others are effective, for example, on respiratory infections or digestive diseases. For many illnesses there is more than one choice.

There is vast ignorance about antibiotics, what they are, how they work, and which ones to use. Sometimes, for infections other than Lyme, the advice given is "Try it and see if it helps." Antibiotic information remains largely unavailable. Nowhere does the public see validation by the health care system of their safety and efficacy. Even those who are most dedicated to getting well may be tempted to settle for "improved" or "better."

ANTIBIOTICS THAT ARE USED FOR LYME DISEASE

Most of the antibiotics used for Lyme disease have long been used for other medical conditions. Tetracycline, Biaxin, and amoxicillin are among the well-known standard antibiotics to treat Lyme disease, although they are used in higher doses than for many other illnesses. Amoxicillin in higher-than-usual amounts can be useful in early disease, and for pregnant women and young children. Not only usually higher doses but a longer time duration has also been found necessary to deal with this spirochete with its extraordinary survival mechanisms for adapting to the immune system and antibiotics. The Burrascano treatment guidelines, "Diagnostic Hints and Treatment for Lyme and Other Tick-Borne Illness," available from the International Lyme and Associated Diseases Society, describe approximately twenty possible antibiotics or antibiotic combinations, with dosages.

Not always are there side effects from Lyme disease antibiotics. Sometimes what appear to be side effect are symptoms of the disease.

For example, Lyme may produce digestive symptoms such as nausea, abdominal pain, or intestinal problems that may or not be caused by the drug. During the months before I was diagnosed, I had bouts of unexplained nausea which disappeared after I started treatment. I was dealing with late-diagnosed Lyme, and my symptoms were so intense that the very mention of side effects appeared ludicrous. I had few or none and always found ways to cope. I ate healthy food and maintained regular meals, sometimes preferring to eat several small meals a day. My blood tests always remained normal, indicating only the presence of Lyme.

Because antibiotics tend to kill "good bacteria" that are needed for digestion as well as killing Lyme bacteria, many during treatment eat live-culture yogurt. Acidophilus pills may be taken as well. In many health food stores enteric-coated acidophilus pills are available in the refrigerated section. The coating prevents the "good" bacteria from being destroyed in the stomach, allowing them to pass through to the intestines where they are needed. Taking acidophilus helps prevent yeast infections that may result from the antibiotic-killing "friendly" bacteria. Occasional yeast infections are treated with over-the-counter medications such as Monistat or GyneLotrimin or a generic version of them.

One of my antibiotics was Biaxin, which I took in combination with Plaquenil. Plaquenil, which allows better intracellular penetration of the Biaxin, is also used for other long-term conditions such as malaria, lupus, and rheumatoid arthritis. It has the very rare, but possible, side effect of causing eye problems and if necessary can be replaced by another medication chosen by the physician. Biaxin sometimes caused a metallic taste in my mouth. But since Biaxin is taken with food, I could eat dinner, have a glass of milk, or brush my teeth and it disappeared. I learned to take it without citrus juices, which act to lower the intracellular acidity, and therefore may interfere with the effectiveness of Biaxin.

Another of my antibiotics, tetracycline, was very effective but sometimes caused nausea. Because that medication is not taken with food, milk, or calcium, I drank an extra glass of water and ate when I could, an hour or so later, and had frequent meals. In general, I was able to avoid stomach discomfort. Occasionally, I "backed off" for a couple of days, as was recommended to me.

Intravenous ceftriaxone (Rocephin) can cause gallstones and, if this happens, can be replaced by another intravenous medication. After being on ceftriaxone for four months, I had a gallbladder test to check for "sludge." The test was normal, showing no gallstones, so I continued the Rocephin for another four months. I've met some people who have reported that "sludge" disappeared when they discontinued ceftriaxone. People who have had their gallbladders removed say that the loss of them was a small price to pay for effective treatment of their disabling disease.

Antibiotics can, and are, switched, according to patient response or discomfort with an antibiotic. Insurance coverage may also enter into choices because some antibiotics are more expensive than others and not all patients have adequate medical insurance coverage. Intravenous antibiotics avoid possible stomach discomfort, but insurance coverage may be a factor.

Response to antibiotics has been found to vary among individuals, and some do better than others on a particular antibiotic. Also, certain ones work better for particular symptoms. I found the intravenous drugs to be useful for the headaches and feelings of intense "head pressure" and general systemic illness that seemed to permeate my whole body. But, in general, I used oral antibiotics, singly or in combination, as most people do. Treatment, as I've said before, requires monitoring and partnership between patient and physician. There is no one protocol that is best for all. Physicians do not necessarily use the same regimens, and all of them tailor the treatment to the clinical picture presented by the patient.

THE INTRAVENOUS LINE AND POSSIBLE PROBLEMS

An infection around the intravenous line can occur, and if signs of inflammation are noted, the line is removed and another one is placed in a different vein. I had no difficulty in my many months of treatment. I took care to follow directions and, in addition, drank plenty of fluids and ate nutritiously. I favored the arm with the IV in it, for example, not using it for heavy lifting, seeing no need to irritate the veins unnecessarily. One of my fellow sufferers, who had neurological problems and was taking an intravenous antibiotic, shoveled her driveway and used a snowblower. Shortly afterward, her line had to be removed and the ceftriaxone replaced by an oral antibiotic.

Those who adhere to the "post-Lyme syndrome" theory of Lyme disease often focus on possible antibiotic side effects, gastrointestinal problems, infections at the site of the intravenous line, and gallstones. Yet, without apparent concern, they continue to put patients on long-term antidepressants, arthritis drugs and other drugs that have no curative value. We hear only about "taking too many antibiotics."

Chapter 11 will give the highlights of research that has been done supporting the need for antibiotic treatment for Lyme disease. I will describe the studies that are used for denying treatment for Lyme disease beyond that of a few weeks. You will see both sides and decide what you would want if you had persisting Lyme disease.

"WHAT DO THE STUDIES SAY?"

THE EXPERTS SPEAK

We know that Lyme disease can persist, and we have our own experiences and the literature that tells us the Lyme spirochete can be difficult to eradicate, and people may remain sick even after months and more. Yet there are those that say they have studies proving there is no chronic Lyme disease. They seem to have their studies and we have ours. How crazy is this anyway?

—LYME PATIENT IN A SUPPORT GROUP

In the previous chapter I told the antibiotic story to provide a guide on how the disease may be treated. The two sides of the Lyme treatment controversy express opposing views of the disease, one saying the disease is always easily treated, and the other that it may persist and become difficult to treat. One would expect that research, as well as clinical experience, would have answered this question long ago, and we would be well on our way to developing more effective antibiotics for treating Lyme disease. However, because the controversy has become a political problem, this has not occurred. The debate continues, and opposition to long-term treatment remains unabated. Those on both sides refer to research studies that appear to support their position.

PROVING ACTIVE INFECTION

As discussed earlier, available blood tests do not confirm continuing infection or even diagnose the disease. And the more serious cases of Lyme are often seronegative, indicating that antibodies are no longer present in the blood, but that does not mean that bacteria are no longer present in the body. Detecting Lyme bacteria by polymerase chain reaction identifies the spirochete and confirms the disease, and finding live spirochetes documents active infection.

RESEARCH ISSUES

With twelve thousand and more studies and papers published on Lyme disease, the expectation would be that they include a plethora of research on treatments to help us document continuing infection. At this time, clinicians who treat patients tailor treatment to the condition of the patient and their clinical experience as they see patients whose knees remain swollen, who continue to experience numbness, and who cannot yet pass the simplest short-term memory tests. Included in this group of Lyme-literate physicians are psychiatrists, neurologists, infectious disease specialists, internists, and others whose training and experience allow them to address the still-unresolved complexities of Lyme disease.

In April 2004, the federal government's Centers for Disease Control announced new awards for Lyme research. The studies in the research were designed to improve understanding of the disease and to examine new methods of testing, prevention, and control rather than to address Lyme disease treatment needs. Grants were given for diagnosis and pathogenesis (biological mechanism) of early Lyme, and one study was funded to advance understanding of the disease's effect on the central nervous system. Another study identifies and evaluates proteins that vary in the cycle between ticks and mammals. A Yale study explores factors that contribute to infection susceptibility and examines characteristics of Lyme disease bacteria that have been crippled by antibiotic treatment. In general, grants are directed toward biochemistry, prevention, and education. They do not help those who are ill.

Dozens of research studies support the persistence of the Lyme spirochete and the benefit from continuing treatment. And both clinical findings and research results demonstrate risks of undertreating the disease. Steere adherents have never refuted studies showing the characteristics of the bacteria that allow them to persist. And their short-term treatment recommendations were put into place long before they produced studies that supported their views that continuing antibiotic treatment is of no value.

RESEARCH STUDIES SUPPORTING
LONGER-TERM TREATMENT

In addition to studies done in the United States, there are those from Italy, Germany, Finland, Sweden, the United Kingdom, Belgium, France, Russia, and Thailand, among others. All demonstrate the ability of the spirochete to persist and the benefit from continuing treatment. One Finnish study described thirteen patients with clinical relapse who had a positive culture, positive PCR, or positive serology, despite having received initial treatment.[1]

Though spirochetes are difficult to detect, they have been cultured, their growth proving active infection. Kenneth Liegner, early in the controversy, said, "Peer-reviewed literature documents the persistence of infection with Borrelia species on biopsy [removal of a tissue sample], culture [growing the bacteria in the laboratory], polymerase chain reaction [PCR] that identifies the spirochete, and autopsy in both animals and humans."[2] Edward Masters, who first identified Lyme disease in Missouri, found spirochetes after continuous high-dose oral therapy.[3]

- Rheinhard Straubinger, a veterinarian, said, "Borrelia burgdorferi disseminate throughout tissue by migration following tick inoculation, producing episodes of acute arthritis, and establishing persistent infection. The spirochete survives antibiotics and disease can be reactivated in immune suppressed animals."[4] These are not treatment studies. What they illustrate is the persistence of the bacteria and possible need for longer-term treatment. We cannot assume that all disease is cured with a few weeks of antibiotic.

- Brian Fallon, director of the Lyme & Tick-Borne Diseases Center at Columbia University, has done neuroimaging studies of brains of those who have Lyme disease. He has used a series of scans over time, combined with scientifically designed cognitive tests. These have shown the changes and improvements that occur with continued treatment that would not occur if spirochetes had been eradicated after a few weeks of treatment.

- Sam Donta has published four articles that document patient improvement with longer-term treatment and better outcomes with longer treatment, showing continued presence of Lyme spirochetes. One of them is a tetracycline treatment study of patients with chronic Lyme disease.[5] A second article discusses the characteristics of late Lyme disease[6] and another gives further information on chronic disease and its treatment.[7] Donta's study on macrolide therapy showed that improvement was related to duration of treatment.[8]

These articles are only a few of those that illustrate the ability of the bacteria and the disease to persist. Alan Macdonald, a pathologist with primary interest in Alzheimer's disease, found Borrelia spirochetes in brain tissue and made slides of the spirochetes including those in cystic form.[9] The fact that the disease could be reactivated after vaccination with the ill-fated Lyme disease vaccine gives further evidence that Lyme bacteria may still exist in the body after treatment.[10]

LEGISLATIVE TESTIMONY ON
PERSISTENCE OF LYME DISEASE

Lyme patients and their doctors testified at the 2004 chronic Lyme disease hearing on the effects on lives caused by long-term Lyme. They were in the position of "proving" that these patients had the disease and remained ill because their disease was not recognized in a timely fashion and their treatment was inadequate. They said the denial of chronic Lyme disease by the Infectious Diseases Society of America was a major factor in their continuing disability.

Although the definitive study on chronic Lyme and the best treatment methods for it has still not been done, there was no doubt that their stories were far from "anecdotal." The immediate purpose of the hearing was to document the problem and provide legislators with information that we already have on the chronic Lyme disease problem. The larger purpose of the hearing was that of gaining acceptance of chronic Lyme disease and laying the groundwork for major public health involvement with the epidemic we now have. The major cause of it is inadequate medical care.

Steven Phillips, an internist who treats chronic Lyme, said at the hearing, "Certainly there are many aspects of Lyme disease which remain highly controversial. And diagnosis and treatment are among the top two. The fact of the matter is that many patients with Lyme disease will relapse despite antibiotic therapy."

Phillips testified on literature published by those who oppose long-term treatment, saying that

> B. Burgdorferi DNA has been detected actually in the muscles of those with so-called post-Lyme fibromyalgia, demonstrating persistence of the organism. And in animal models, despite 30 days of Amoxicillin, or Doxycycline, eradication of the organism was not achieved. When they've

expanded these studies to include not only Amoxicillin and Doxycycline but also Azithromycin and intravenous ceftri-axone at comparable human doses for 30 days, the same thing happened. The bacteria was [sic] not eliminated from these animals.

He said 30 percent of the patients remained seropositive for PCR despite multiple courses of traditional short-term treatment.[11]

He testified that authors of articles published by those who treat the disease short term found live Bb spirochetes in the eye, heart, spleen, lymph nodes, ligaments, and joints, despite antibiotics. Live spirochetes were cultured in blood and other organs. "Here they found it in the heart in a fatal case of Lyme disease from Lyme carditis, despite, quote, unquote adequate treatment." Phillips offered seventy-one references that included many different authors.[12]

Brian Fallon testified on neuropsychiatric aspects of the disease, saying, "I think there are a number of general aspects of Lyme disease that cause distress and confusion. One is that symptoms fluctu-ate. Patients are often worse on some days, better on others. That confuses parents, school systems, employers, spouses. It's a difficult aspect of this illness." He spoke of the well-known laboratory test-ing problem with results that often vary, depending on the test, the laboratory, and the stage of the illness. He explained the many pos-sible neurological symptoms of Lyme, and how to differentiate them from psychiatric illness.

Fallon spoke of a 1998 study on children done by Steere and his group, saying that of eighty-six children who had been treated for Lyme disease, twelve had neurocognitive problems. He then described his Columbia study that included children whose diagnosis was delayed and who had problems with working memory and the processing of au-ditory and visual input after being given an average of 2.3 months of in-travenous antibiotics and 7.5 months of oral antibiotics.[13]

Fallon said, "Finally, I just want to emphasize that children are suffering in the school systems. They look like they're inattentive, unmotivated, disorganized and confused. They fall asleep in class. They may look good, even on bad days. Children may function better on some days. It drives parents and teachers crazy." He recommended that "a state-wide educational update on Lyme disease should be considered for all teachers, principals, and special ed coordinators in Connecticut" and concluded by saying,

> What academic Lyme experts write in journals or state from podiums may differ from what they do with their own patients. And that's because the practice of clinical medicine remains an art in which medical care is individualized for each patient. We work with uncertainty much of the time and we learn from our patients and from the journals. So, in the face of insufficient medical knowledge, we need to keep an open mind. Doctors need freedom to practice. And definitive practice guidelines, regardless of who publishes them should not be made until far more research is completed.[14]

Lyme patients applauded. They could not agree more. An open mind and freedom to practice medicine according to physicians' best judgment is exactly what those in the Lyme community, the organizations, patients, and physicians, are asking. We cannot have lockstep denial of treatment for persistent Lyme disease.

STUDIES DENYING PERSISTING INFECTION

Problems seen with research denying chronic Lyme disease have been identified and published in physician response letters to the *New England Journal of Medicine* and others. Problematic design, the unreliability of Lyme disease tests, and other factors have undermined public acceptance of study results. The problems fall into the following categories:

- The sample was too small.
- The sample was poorly selected.
- The treatment regimen was too short.
- The wrong antibiotic was used.
- Conclusions are not supported by evidence.
- Studies appear designed to support a predetermined outcome.

THE SEA CHANGE THAT OCCURRED IN 1993

Before 1993, a number of Lyme disease physicians, who have since published extensively denying chronic Lyme disease, acknowledged possible persistence of Lyme disease. Among them are Allen Steere, who first identified Lyme disease at Yale University and is now professor of medicine at Harvard; Mark Klempner, formerly at the New England Medical Center and who is now associate provost for research at Boston Univerity; and Robert Shoen, a rheumatologist formerly at Yale who worked with Steere and is now affiliated with New York Medical College in Valhalla, New York. Until 1992, papers by Steere, Shoen, and other IDSA physicians acknowledged chronic Lyme disease and possible need for re-treatment.

Steere commented in the *New England Journal of Medicine*, saying in the abstract, "Treatment with appropriate antibiotics is usually curative, but longer courses of therapy are often needed for later in the illness, and some patients may not respond."[15] Other publications, also written by IDSA physicians, gave the same message. For example, Robert Schoen said, "Later stages of the illness are frequently more difficult to treat, requiring prolonged oral or intravenous antibiotic therapy.[16] In 1992 Mark Klempner's name was included in an article reporting that live spirochetes can be recovered long after initial infection even from antibiotic-treated patients, "indicating that it resists eradication by host defense mechanisms and antibiotics."[17] These are representative of a number of articles published in earlier years indicating that the disease is not always easily cured.

Steere was among the researchers reporting on a study of twenty-seven patients saying, "Months to years after the initial infection with B. burgdorferi, patients with Lyme disease may have chronic encephalopathy, polyneuropathy, or less commonly, leukoencephalitis [inflammation of the white matter of the brain]. These abnormalities usually improve with antibiotic therapy." The study reported that after six months, more than one third of the patients had relapsed or were no better. In addition, more than half had previously received antibiotic treatment thought to be appropriate for their stage of the disease and still had progression of their disease. The likely reason for relapse is "failure to completely eradicate the spirochete completely with a two–week course of intravenous ceftriaxone therapy." Hypothesized is that irreversible damage to the nervous system may have occurred.[18]

By the time of the 1993 congressional hearing on Lyme disease (see Chapter 7), chaired by Senator Edward Kennedy, their position had changed. This is when the controversy on treating Lyme disease first became evident. Steere presented his research on Lyme disease and showed, as an example, a patient who had recovered from the disease. Joseph Burrascano described Lyme disease as a complex disease that is not easily treated and accused Steere researchers of conflicts of interest. And the struggle between the two camps has continued ever since.

CHANGE IN MEDICAL TEXTBOOK INFORMATION

Conn's Current Therapy is a classic medical textbook that was first published in 1949, and W. B. Saunders Company publishes a new edition annually. As late as 1997, the section on Lyme disease was written by Joseph Burrascano, the physician who faced investigation in 2000 for overtreating Lyme. In 1998, it was written by Allen Steere with a dif-

ferent opinion, and this characterization of the disease in *Conn's Current Therapy* has been printed ever since.

In 2000, a clear description of differences was published in *Pediatrics,* the official journal of the American Academy of Pediatrics.

The two camps are clearly outlined in two consecutive editions of *Conn's Current Therapy.*

In the 1997 edition, Joseph J. Burrascano, Jr., MD, (a community-based physician) gives his method of diagnosing and treating Lyme disease. Dr. Burrascano states that Lyme disease "is an extremely complex illness that is still poorly understood." He notes that fewer than 50 percent of patients with Lyme disease present with the classic rash— erythema migrans. "The diagnosis of Lyme disease is made on clinical grounds including a response to empiric antibiotics and no currently available laboratory test is definitive. Parenteral (intravenous) therapy is recommended for patients with persistent symptoms unresponsive to oral therapy and for patients with severe disease. Management of Lyme disease is a "therapeutic alliance between the physician and the patient."

In the 1998 edition of *Conn's Current Therapy*, Allen C. Steere (an academic-based physician) gives his method of diagnosing and treating Lyme disease. Dr. Steere states that >75 percent of patients with Lyme disease present with erythema migrans. The other patients present with objective signs involving the nervous system, heart or joints. "Serologic (blood) testing is the most practical laboratory aid to diagnosis." To diagnose Lyme disease with nervous system, heart or joint involvement, Borrelia burgdorferi serology should be positive. Lyme disease can usually be

treated successfully with oral antibiotics, except neurological disease, which usually requires intravenous therapy.[19]

Lyme organizations and patients disagree with the Steere position on
the value of diagnosis by testing and his view of apparently problem-
free treatment. Their experience correlates with information provided
in the Burrascano statement of 1997. It is this split within the medical
world that helps deny medical care for Lyme for those whose disease is
not easily treated.

STUDIES DENYING THE EXISTENCE OF CHRONIC LYME DISEASE

On July 12, 2001, the *New England Journal of Medicine* published a
short–term study on a limited number of patients. It was a ninety-day
time duration on patients who had already failed the thirty-day treatment. In reality it was not a study on chronic disease. It was a short-
term study, with an antibiotic regimen deemed inadequate by those who
treat chronic Lyme disease. Whether the disease was early or late diagnosed remained a question. However, this study continues to be used in
denying long-term Lyme disease. No reason was given for selecting the
short-term ninety-day treatment plan. Many people require far longer
to resolve their symptoms.

With Mark Klempner as the lead author, 129 patients were enrolled in the study and divided into two groups, 78 having a positive
Lyme test and 51 with a negative test. Those in both groups received
either a placebo or thirty days of intravenous ceftriaxone followed by
sixty days of oral doxycycline. The studies were discontinued after the
first 107 patients because data of the 129 patients indicated that it
was highly unlikely that a significant difference in treatment efficacy
between the two groups would be observed with the full enrollment.
The reason given for terminating the study was that there were no
significant differences in outcomes with prolonged antibiotic treatment as compared with a placebo.

For a patient to be enrolled in the study, symptoms had to have appeared within six months after the initial infection and to have persisted for at least six months but less than twelve years. Data was collected by questionnaires. Those with a positive PCR test were excluded from the study, although that requirement was never satisfactorily explained. When questioned, Klempner said he found no positive PCRs. No mention was made of Herxheimer responses that may occur when the spirochete reacts to the antibiotic and affect patient perception of the severity of symptoms. The studies on the patient groups were publicized nationwide in major media outlets, including the *New York Times*. No subsequent study has yet addressed the questions raised by this one.

The suffering that is experienced by those with Lyme disease was acknowledged. "The effect of chronic Lyme disease on the health-related quality of life was substantial in both groups," said Klempner. "The deficits in physical health status as measured. . . were equivalent to those with congestive heart failure or osteoarthritis." And he added, "Chronic pain was an important contributor to the impairment of physical health."[20]

DURATION OF ANTIBIOTICS AND OUTCOME

As principal investigator, Gary Wormser did a treatment study of 180 patients with the erythema migrans rash. The protocols were ten days of doxycycline, with or without a single intravenous dose of ceftriaxone, or twenty days of oral doxycycline. Results were assessed at twenty days, three months, twelve months, and thirty months.

No benefit was shown with prolonged treatment except that patients who were given doxycycline plus ceftriaxone had diarrhea more often than patients given doxycycline alone. Conclusions were made that extending treatment with doxycycline from ten to twenty days or adding one dose of ceftriaxone to the beginning of a ten-day course of treatment did not enhance therapeutic efficacy in regard to the erythema migrans rash. "Objective evidence of treatment failure was extremely rare."[21]

The number of patients, 180, would not seem enough to dictate policy decisions and assure patient safety, and the spread between ten and twenty days of treatment would also seem too short to make major decisions on limiting treatment for early Lyme disease. A single-dose intravenous ceftriaxone appears almost irrelevant in making treatment decisions. In addition, success is measured in terms of the disappearance of the rash, a criterion that is inadequate in determining whether the spirochetes have been eliminated.

Nevertheless, this study is used as reference for decisions made to limit the duration of antibiotics. In addition, the rash may appear later. It may not be possible to determine that this was early Lyme disease. Finally, the timeframe is not long enough to show possible differences, and the disappearance of the rash does not indicate the disease is cured.

Andrea Gaito, past president of the International Lyme and Associated Diseases Society, critiqued the study by saying that over 50 percent of the subjects in each of the study groups were subsequently re-treated with a second course of antibiotics for other conditions. She reported that these unrelated illnesses occurred in previously ultra-healthy groups. "Over half of the patients were retreated in the ensuing 30 months with antibiotics under the guise of other illnesses."[22]

GIVING PREVENTIVE ANTIBIOTICS

Eugene Shapiro said in the *New England Journal of Medicine* that "persons bitten by a deer tick should not routinely receive antimicrobial chemoprophylaxis [preventive antibiotics]," listing costs, adverse effects, and efficacy of antimicrobial prophylaxis. "It may be reasonable to administer doxycycline in areas where the incidence of Lyme is high and when the tick is a nymphal deer tick that is at least partially engorged with blood . . . if chemoprophylaxis is chosen, only a single dose of doxycycline should be administered."[23]

Shapiro referenced a study done with Robert Nadelman as the principal investigator. Nadelman found that with a single dose of doxycycline administered, the efficacy was 87 percent. Objective ex-

tracutaneous signs of Lyme disease did not appear in these subjects and there were no asymptomatic seroconversions, meaning that they developed no signs of Lyme other than the rash, and their Lyme disease tests did not become positive.[24]

Many who discover a deer tick that is as small as a poppy seed or less will not know whether the tick is a nymph or an adult, or whether or not it is engorged. They will not know how long it was attached, or that the rash represents early disease. Efficacy rate of 87 percent may not be acceptable to the public.

OTHER STUDIES DENYING CHRONIC LYME DISEASE

Nancy Shadick studied 186 patients on Nantucket who had had Lyme disease in the past, and 167 who had not. The study was funded by the National Institutes of Health, with follow-up at six years. Using the Nantucket census, a survey was mailed to six thousand residents over the age of 17, and participants were selected from those who responded as determined by criteria.

Results were obtained by patient responses to a one-page written survey. Those with a history of Lyme disease reported no more musculoskeletal, neurological, or neurocognitive abnormalities than did the healthy controls. Although people had generally recovered, the questionnaires revealed that many of the participants who had had Lyme reported not being able to perform daily tasks without difficulties such as pain. The conclusion was made: "Because persons with previous Lyme disease exhibited no sequalae on physical examination and neurocognitive tests a mean of 6.0 years after infection, musculoskeletal and neurocognitve outcomes seem to be favorable. However, long-term impairment of functional status can occur."[25]

Neurologists criticized the measurement scale that was used and noted no treatment component in the study. Patients questioned that "healthy" people have musculoskeletal, neurological, or neurocognitive abnormalities.

Robert Kalish evaluated eighty-four patients with Lyme disease in

a ten- to twenty-year follow-up study, concluding that residual symptoms were a result of "post-Lyme syndrome," not active infection. "These patients were functioning relatively well, despite neurocognitive, pain or fatigue syndromes." He said the pathogenesis was unclear and hypothesized regarding stressful emotional events as a cause. "Perhaps diffuse or prolonged CNS [central nervous system] infection with B. burgdorferi in susceptible people triggers immunologic or neurohormonal processes that perpetuate this post infectious syndrome. However, we do not know whether this is a direct effect of CNS infection or an indirect effect of a particularly stressful event."[26]

Always, in studies done by those who opposed more than short-term treatment, the goal appears to be that of shortening treatment rather than reducing possible risk for those who are bitten by an infected deer tick.

Physicians who do not agree that active infection may persist after short-term treatment cite reasons for denying treatment by saying that there is no proof of active infection, risk of antibiotic side effects, possible infections with intravenous infusions, and gallstones, but they do acknowledge that antibiotics for Lyme do not produce Lyme-resistant bacteria. As I said earlier, Lyme victims are dead-end hosts that do not transmit the disease to others. They even contact legislators to express opposition to legislation that would allow medical treatment for persistent Lyme disease. I quote from one of them.

On June 28, 2005, Walter Stamm, the IDSA president, wrote to Governor Edward G. Rendell of Pennsylvania, speaking of no benefit and possible harm from longer-term antibiotics for Lyme disease. Two years later, on August 7, 2007, Dr. Henry Mazur, then the president of IDSA, affirmed in a two-page letter to the Honorable Jon S. Corzine, chairman of the Health and Human Services Committee of the National Governors Association in Washington, D.C., that antibiotics for Lyme do not produce Lyme-resistant bacteria. In the first paragraph he said,

I write on behalf of the Infectious Diseases Society of America [IDSA] to bring to the National Governors Association [NGA] attention [to] problematic Lyme disease legislation that has been introduced in several states. In making NGA aware of these legislative efforts, many of which are well-intentioned, but therapeutically dangerous, our primary concern is to ensure the best quality in patient care and to protect the public's health and safety. To this end, we believe it is critically important that you be fully apprised of the widespread consensus within the medical and scientific community about the appropriate treatment for Lyme disease, as well as the medical community's concerns about unproven, potentially harmful treatments for so called "chronic Lyme disease" that are advocated by a small group of physicians.

WHAT ABOUT A VACCINE FOR LYME DISEASE?

Chapter 12 will discuss the failed Lyme disease vaccine that showed such promise that few questioned its possible side effects. It was developed by those who oppose long-term treatment, and the studies associated with its development reflected some of the same problems for the public as those that are used to limit treatment for Lyme disease.

"WHATEVER HAPPENED TO THE LYME VACCINE?"

LESSONS LEARNED ABOUT MEDICAL RESEARCH

I thought there was a vaccine for this disease. I know people who had it, but when I asked my doctor he said there is no vaccine for Lyme.

—CITIZEN WHO CALLED HER TOWN'S
SENIOR CENTER FOR A FLU SHOT

W ith Lyme disease becoming more prevalent every year, the market for a preventive vaccine seemed favorable, and there was no reason to expect that it would fail. The Lymerix vaccine was developed by many of the same well-funded physicians who obstruct progress in medical care by maintaining that Lyme is overdiagnosed and overtreated, and saying there is no such thing as chronic Lyme disease. They published the problematic studies that were described in the preceding chapter. One might ask, as many did, "If this infection is always so easily treated that even heart block is cured within a few weeks, why is the need for a vaccine so urgent?"

Soon after its introduction, the question of need became irrelevant. The Lymerix vaccine was a disaster almost from the start. Many

drugs, later found to be harmful, remain on the market for a number of years before they are withdrawn, even when the risk of taking them appears unacceptable or the drugs are discovered to be ineffective. The Lyme disease vaccine lasted less than two years.

The Revolving Door in Medical Research

The Food and Drug Administration approves new drugs that are developed by pharmaceutical companies. The agency is underfunded and understaffed, lacking resources to do much of its own research, so studies on new products are often done by the companies that manufacture the drug. Scientists and consultants working for the FDA come from the corporate world and later rejoin pharmaceutical companies where the pay is far better than in the government agency.

With urgency to move new medications to market, objectivity can be compromised. Large amounts of money are involved over long periods of time, and conflicts of interest become possible. The web of connections among the interested parties can be difficult to penetrate, as it was in development of the Lymerix vaccine. Testimony on this was presented at the Albany, New York, chronic Lyme disease hearing by Pamela Weintraub, a science journalist, who researched and cross-referenced every relevant patent and grant to members of five decision-making regulatory bodies connected with the vaccine:

> I did not find evidence of conspiracy amidst my thousand points of data, nor did I find any crime. Instead, as I conducted my research, I found what is almost mundane. An appearance of conflict of interest, in which decisions are made by committees on Lyme disease policy that had the potential to benefit the intellectual property of some of the committee members, their employers, or the companies they received grants from or consulted for. Such conflicts are business as usual in the United States today and have been reported and validated across many other fields of

medicine. I can report, based on my research, that Lyme disease joins the crowd.[1]

As others have noted, the apparent conflict of interest, which has become increasingly evident in the world of science, began in 1980 with the passage of the Bayh/Dole Act, known as the Dole Law. In her testimony Weintraub says, "This Act enables universities and individuals to patent federally funded research results for their own profit. The business model of the relevant patents [for Lyme disease] turns out to be a series of increasingly complex vaccines and related test kits, with a different test kit to diagnose Lyme disease for each version of the vaccine."

Marcia Angell, the former editor of the prestigious *New England Journal of Medicine*, describes the process of how drugs are now brought to market, including the use of universities for pharmaceutical company research, a system that by its design works to interfere with objectivity and includes legions of lawyers that stretch out government-granted marketing rights for years.[2]

EFFECT ON MEDICAL CARE FOR LYME

It seemed that the vaccine might help to resolve the diagnosis and treatment controversy that makes every tick bite a matter of concern. Managed health companies act to restrict medical care for many illnesses other than Lyme. For example, they approve coverage for procedures, decide what drugs are allowed for treating specified medical conditions, and tell you how many days in the hospital will be permitted. But, for Lyme, a disease that has been controlled in almost every aspect by a very few physicians, this has been a special problem. It is often an intracellular disease, where spirochetes are located inside cells and are not recognized by the immune system, and this requires physician-prescribed antibiotics for its cure. The length of time necessary to eradicate the infection cannot be predetermined, and arbitrary cut-off has no scientific basis. Yet doctors who provide necessary medical services continue to be

harassed and investigated by insurance companies and IDSA-controlled state medical boards. As mentioned in Chapter 11, in 2007 the Infectious Diseases Society of America president wrote the New Jersey governor warning against passing legislation that would protect medical care and insurance coverage for Lyme disease.

It is an incredible occurrence for a medical group to advocate against insurance coverage for patients. This does not happen for alternative medicine, with its unproven herbs and procedures, or with antibiotics for other conditions. It's only about common, everyday, often inexpensive, antibiotics that are used for treating Lyme disease.

To show you how aggressively the physicians who write the IDSA's Lyme policy protect their position, at least two other letters are known to have appeared earlier opposing legislation for medical coverage. On June 28, 2005, Governor Edward Rendell of Pennsylvania received a letter with the same message from the IDSA president when legislative action was proposed for that state. And on August 18, 2005, Walter Stamm, president of the IDSA, wrote to the Honorable Joe Barton, chairman of the Committee on Energy and Commerce, advocating against a proposed Lyme disease education bill and a bill that would create a tick-borne diseases advisory committee.

In response, on August 26, 2007, the president of the Canadian Lyme Disease Foundation wrote his own letter to Governor Jon Corzine of New Jersey, chairman of the Health and Human Services Committee of the National Governors Association. He described the role of nationalized medical care on restricting medical treatment in Canada, and, since far more is done here, Canada's reliance on U.S. medical research, including the IDSA's guidelines for Lyme disease. He explained the harm they are doing to those in Canada with Lyme disease, saying, "The IDSA guidelines have done more harm to people throughout North America than any other medical guidelines we are aware of."

In his letter he asked, "If the IDSA is that confident in their recommended testing protocol, how possibly could Lyme bacteria be showing up in the numbers it is in these other diseases (Alzheimer's, Multiple Sclerosis, Colitis, Crohn's disease and many others)." He said:

> Until proper post mortem, and multiple live tissue studies per victim, employing all testing technology available, is done on victims of those several diseases linked to Borrelia burgdorferi, the bacteria that cause Lyme disease, very little can be said about present testing accuracy, prevalence, what symptoms can be attributed to chronic Lyme disease, and what treatment methods are effective. This makes the entire IDSA document premature and not worthy of a health care guideline.[3]

Those in the Lyme community would agree. We don't have appropriate information that allows such dogmatic guidelines. Physicians and patients are on the front lines and need to be allowed to access information that we do have for better diagnosis and treatment. Especially, the public and physicians should know about disease that has progressed beyond the early stage. Both physicians and patients must be free to make decisions according to need and judgment, as they do for other diseases.

THE LYMERIX VACCINE

The vaccine did nothing to resolve the Lyme controversy. For some Lyme patients, their problems increased. When it was introduced to the public in January 1999, many who had barely heard of Lyme disease rushed to their physicians to get the shots. Promotion was intense. During the first year 1.4 million doses of it were delivered, and it generated $40 million in sales. Those who received the vaccine were saying, "Now I won't have to worry about Lyme disease."

It was rushed to market because of the soaring numbers of people with Lyme disease. No warnings were given to either physicians or the public about possible adverse events, other than possible irritation at the injection site. Although some physicians held back, waiting for more information, both the public and their physicians were already primed to accept the shots. We needed a means to prevent the disease besides relying on checking for ticks every time we went outdoors beyond the edges of our lawns. We have vaccines for smallpox, polio, measles, the human papillovirus, so why not Lyme disease?

For researchers, universities, health departments, and pharmaceutical companies, the public need for a vaccine offered unparalleled opportunity that included government funding. The Dole Law gave universities, small businesses, and nonprofit organizations intellectual property control of the inventions that resulted from federal government-funded research. It also allowed the funding agency, under certain conditions, to grant additional licenses to other applicants. With the passage of the 1980 Dole Law, new partnerships became possible among universities, funding agencies, and corporations. Universities were allowed to share in profits generated from products developed from their research. Licensing, venture capital, contract research, and corporate technical relations are among the ways that universities interact with the private sector.

GlaxoSmithKline developed the Lymerix vaccine in partnership with Yale, and the trials were directed by Allen Steere. At least two other drug companies, along with health departments, scientists, and physicians, had shares in the almost-guaranteed success of this product. The relationships were complex but beneficial to all who participated in bringing the vaccine to market.

In order to create a vaccine for the rapidly growing disease, a case definition of Lyme first had to be developed. Therefore, in 1994, members of the CDC and researchers met in Fort Collins, Colorado, and decided to use the surveillance standard, the so-called Dearborn criteria, to define Lyme disease. These criteria affirmed the two-tiered testing system, the ELISA, to be followed by the (also problematic)

Western blot that contained five positive bands, the definition used to-day that severely restricts acceptance of the diagnosis of Lyme disease.

The Western blot test separates the spirochete's proteins electrically. They are blotted onto paper and, when exposed to the patient's blood serum and an enzyme solution, form bands. If antibodies have not formed, no markings (bands) indicating exposure to Lyme disease will appear. Bands may appear early, late, or not at all. Some of the protein bands appear more frequently than others. As explained in Chapter 5, however, having no positive bands does not mean you don't have Lyme disease.

Pamela Weintraub's research revealed that two of the bands most indicative of Lyme disease, the Osp A and Osp B, were removed from surveillance criteria, to be reserved for use in vaccine development. Osp A was planned for use in the Lymerix vaccine, with Osp B reserved for the next generation of vaccine trials. Removing two bands most indicative of Lyme from the surveillance criteria, in the minds of many, constitutes fraud.

Lymerix was not a "live vaccine," and as a result, without information to the contrary, most considered it safe. No spirochetes, living or dead, were injected. The substance used was Osp A, an outer surface protein of the spirochete that served as the antigen (resulting in antibody formation to fight infection). Injecting the antigen from the Borrelia burgdorferi bacteria provoked a protective immune response against the disease.

By using Osp A in the vaccine to stimulate antibody production, though, subsequent Western blots showed this positive band in those who were vaccinated. Since people who received the shots were injected with the antigen Osp A, if they got Lyme in the future, this band would indicate that they had disease. Therefore, it became irrelevant as a diagnostic tool. Regardless of whether or not people were bit by an infected tick, the test result would be positive and had to be discounted. And since both the ELISA and Western blot were already known as unreliable, excluding Osp A and Osp B for use in vaccine development presented a further obstacle in diagnosing this many-faceted disease.

STUDY DESIGN

Eleven thousand people were enrolled in the study that preceded the vaccine's introduction to the public in 1999, with half receiving the vaccine and the other half a placebo, or "sugar pill." People with Lyme disease within the past three months were excluded from participating in the study trial; those with past Lyme disease were not. It was possible that they had been undertreated, in accord with the overtreated school of thought espoused by the vaccine researchers. They could still have had the disease when they were injected with Lymerix. The assumption could well have been made that they were cured.

The study design called for healthy enrollees, although it was reported that more than two thousand had prior history of musculoskeletal or neurological disorders, making possible the conclusion that vaccine failures could be attributed to preexisting medical conditions other than new or persisting Lyme disease. The vaccine trial lasted only eighteen months, a matter of concern to some because late-appearing problems might be missed, since in Lyme disease symptoms often appear far distant from the initial infection. Heart, nerve, muscle, and other organs may appear healthy, but in fact, damage has occurred.

Three doses of vaccine were given, the second administered one month after the first, and the third dose given at the end of one year. Consideration was being given to making the vaccine available to pediatric patients as well as the adult population.

INITIAL RESULTS AND STUDY DESIGN QUESTIONS

Trial results, reported at FDA meetings and in scientific literature, showed the vaccine was 76 percent effective in preventing Lyme disease after all three shots had been given. Critics said that the lack of acceptable Lyme tests and the narrow definition of the disease by researchers who designed the vaccine (including positive ELISA and Western blot tests, rash, arthritis occurring in area endemic for Lyme), made assessment of the vaccine's effectiveness questionable from the beginning.

Also not addressed in these trials were possible coinfections with other tick-borne diseases such as ehrlichiosis, babesiosis, and bartonella that may accompany Lyme disease, or the many possible strains of the Borrelia spirochete. Participants may have had in their bodies microorganisms of these diseases as well as Lyme.

No follow-up was planned beyond one year after the participants received the three shots, far too short a time, in the minds of many, to assess long-term results. Not addressed was the possible need for booster shots, although it was known that the vaccine's immunological benefits declined rapidly. If the Lymerix studies had continued before its introduction to the public, some of these questions would undoubtedly have been considered.

PROBLEMS OCCURRING DURING THE TRIALS BEFORE INTRODUCTION TO THE PUBLIC

The problems that surfaced with the Lymerix vaccine during the trials appeared to mirror those of previous studies that denied persisting Lyme disease. For example, the Klempner studies published in 2000 were done on a limited number of people for a duration of only three months, with drugs deemed inadequate by those who are experienced in treating the disease. Nevertheless, the authors claimed that it proved that no benefit accrued from continuing treatment.

Prior to vaccination, enrollees could have had symptomatic, or asymptomatic, chronic Lyme. Because researchers involved in the study did not accept the diagnosis of persisting or chronic Lyme, this possibility could not be considered in assessing success of the vaccine.

Adverse events could not be adequately identified and, when they occurred, were not always accepted for what they were. This was made more possible because we don't have a test that assured (1) that the subjects no longer had Lyme or (2) that they didn't have undiagnosed

Lyme. The bottom line was that without knowing the health status of the enrollees, the difficulty of assessing benefit and risks of a mass-introduced vaccine could only be problematic. Subjects with adverse events after taking the vaccine found themselves in a situation similar to that of those with chronic Lyme disease whose diagnosis is denied. Hundreds turned to the FDA and then to their lawyers. At least four lawsuits are known to have been filed before the vaccine was even introduced to the public.

Lyme-literate physicians and scientists expressed concerns before the vaccine became available. The research was a badly organized and run effort, but there was nothing anyone could do if it was approved by the FDA. A few FDA officials expressed concern, but behind the new product was a network of powerful groups that included the U.S. Centers for Disease Control.

Adverse Reactions Following Introduction of the Vaccine to the Public

The vaccine was approved in December 1998 and introduced to the public in January 1999. Reports of illness from the vaccine appeared soon after it came on the market. During the first year 298 adverse reactions were received, with 10 percent of the participants having symptoms of chronic arthritis. Often, symptoms were not acknowledged by doctors who were uninformed about the disease and could not believe that an approved vaccine could cause such problems, certainly not ones that could be incurable and persist for life.

The research design did not address adequately the adverse effects that might occur as a result of receiving the vaccine. For example, when problems were reported, researchers had no reporting category for Bell's palsy, a facial nerve condition that is a frequent symptom of Lyme. Neurological problems can be multiple and variable, from headaches to memory loss, numbness, fatigue, cognitive impairment, and more. Symptoms might not be accepted without a positive spinal tap, a test that seldom provides information on Lyme, even with active infection. Although most people took the vaccine without ill effects, and were comfortable with the assumption that they were now protected from Lyme disease, this favorable result could not be assured for all.

No information was provided on how long the protection might last. It was known to be limited and booster shots would be required. Protection was incomplete and did not replace other preventive measures, such as checking for ticks.

Sam Donta reported on a study of his patients who had been given the vaccine and concluded,

> The Lyme Osp A vaccine appears to be reactivating symptoms [arthritis and neurological symptoms] characteristic of chronic Lyme disease. Individuals without known prior infection with B. burgdorferi who had vaccine-assisted reactions had evidence of prior infection by Western blot analyses. As the numbers of reactions among vaccine recipients appears to be increasing, and the magnitude of this problem is yet to be delineated, it would seem appropriate to withhold the vaccine with a prior history of Lyme disease and/or have patients tested with a sensitive Western blot prior to receiving the vaccine. [4]

Vaccine failures could be hard to determine. For it to be counted as a failure (in protecting against Lyme disease) the enrollee had to meet the strict CDC Lyme disease case reporting definition that was discussed in Chapter 5 on diagnosing Lyme disease (positive ELISA and Western blot tests with five positive bands). An erythema migrans rash alone might not qualify in documenting a vaccine failure. A photograph might also be required. The Lyme Disease Foundation reported that documents, obtained later, revealed that criteria used for some of the adverse events were not always consistent, especially neurological symptoms. The Freedom of Information Act allows access to some internal documents. Reporting problems continued to shadow the credibility of the vaccine.

The *New York Times* reported in 2000,

> The Food and Drug Administration said 500 cases [adverse events resulting from taking the shots] have been reported from among the more than one million vaccine doses SmithKlineBeecham [now GlaxoSmithKline] says it has sold. Of the 500 cases, the agency said 45 were considered serious, which means an individual needed hospitalization, or developed a life-threatening illness or a permanent disability.[5]

The same news story told the experience of a New Jersey hospice nurse. "A week after the second of three shots required for immunization she found herself in unbearable pain, and within months, she was so stiff and suffering such pain in her chest and arms that she could barely move for hours in the morning." Her husband developed the same form of arthritis that afflicted his wife.

Reports continued to come from people who became ill, sometimes after only one dose, or sometimes two doses, of the vaccine. Other press stories followed, such as that of two women who developed a severe and untreatable form of arthritis after taking the vaccine.[6] Most people who took the shot had no side effects, but those who became permanently ill faced problems they could not have imagined. Published stories showed ill effects so catastrophic that it was hard to believe that they could be due to the vaccine.

Reported symptoms were likely to be attributed to something else, exactly as symptoms of chronic Lyme disease are often ascribed to, for example, multiple sclerosis, fibromyalgia, or psychosomatic illness. Frequently, doctors involved in the study were reported to be dismissive of symptoms, not following up promptly and fairly. Doctors of patients who took the vaccine after its approval could often not understand the symptoms, or associate them with the vaccine.

CLASS ACTION LAWSUITS FILED

Within months, continuing reports of adverse events could not be ignored. Individual and class action suits were filed, with more in
progress. The cases addressed efficacy, duration of protection, safety,
and other issues, including the design that did not address possible
presence of other tick-borne infections. Most important of all, a
major cause of permanent, disabling, catastrophic side effects was
uncovered.

Stephen Sheller, of Sheller, Ludwig, and Badey in Pennsylvania,
filed one of the lawsuits (No. 99–10423) representing 350 clients
who were harmed by Lymerix.

> The class [class action suit] is believed to be comprised of
> tens, if not hundreds, of thousands of persons, and is
> therefore so numerous that joinder [a legal term meaning
> inclusion of additional parties and issues] of all members
> is impracticable. At the same time, the value of the relief
> sought herein for each member of the class is too little to
> justify individual legal action on behalf of all members of
> the class.

Regarding efficacy, the suit said,

> The commercial, the literature and news reports have
> cited an 80 percent efficacy rate in preventing "definite"
> and "asymptomatic" Lyme disease. However, if you in-
> clude the category of "possible" Lyme disease as well, the
> overall efficacy rate is 69 percent. If you include the cat-
> egory of "unconfirmed" Lyme disease, in which the vac-
> cine has negative efficacy, or some percentage of those
> cases, the efficacy rate is even lower, closer to 50 percent.

The reported efficacy figures depend upon a semantic/ definitional game—by creating different categories of vaccines for the statistics SmithKline [sic] has hidden the overall poor efficacy of the this vaccine.

The suit reported that these results occurred after three shots, but the efficacy rate one year after the third shot has been given falls to nearly what it was after only two shots.

A MAJOR CULPRIT IN ADVERSE REACTIONS TO THE LYME VACCINE IS FOUND

The lawsuit claimed, "Twenty-one common issues and questions of law and fact existing among the Class members as against Defendant with respect to Lymerix" were presented. First on the list was the problem with the Osp A, the outer surface protein of the spirochete used as the antigen.

It said, "Whether Lymerix is unreasonably dangerous as designed, manufactured, marketed, and sold in that it utilizes Osp A as its primary active component for immunological efficacy although a substantial portion of the general population, estimated to be as high as thirty percent (30 percent) are of a specific genetic type known as HLA-DR4+ [sic]." The complaint continues that it "results in their significantly higher predisposition for the onset of treatment-resistant Lyme Arthritis when exposed to Osp A, and thus, places them at a high risk for developing treatment-resistant Lyme arthritis upon taking Lymerix."

With 30 percent of the population having this genetic marker, and without this knowledge prior to taking the vaccine, a major portion of the population faced risk from taking it, even a single dose.

Other autoimmune diseases were triggered by the vaccine, Dr. Fein says it triggers lupus, B27 arthritis, MS, Parkinsonian features, and so forth.

WHAT RESEARCHERS KNEW

Members of the FDA panel had expressed misgivings before approving Lymerix, but the need to bring it to market was urgent. Concerns about the Osp A protein and the HLA-DR4 gene were known, that those carrying this gene may develop what is considered an autoimmune response. This leads to incurable arthritis and other symptoms of Lyme disease. Later documents revealed that this link was discussed at the May 1998 meeting of the FDA advisory panel that reviewed the clinical trials conducted by GlaxoSmithKline, which produced the vaccine, to demonstrate its safety.

Edward Silverman, a reporter, said that "in October 1998, patients participating in a clinical trial were asked to sign papers indicating that a 'theoretical possibility' existed that the vaccine might cause arthritis in genetically susceptible individuals." This information came from documents obtained by the *Star Ledger*.[7] Although those in the trial before its approval signed a paper, those taking the vaccine after its approval and their doctors were not told.

Allen Steere, in an article in the July 1998 *Science,* two months after he recommended that the FDA approve the vaccine (in December 1998), in which he was interviewed (and which was referenced in the *Star Ledger*), noted that the genetic link "is an issue of concern . . . ongoing surveillance will be important." Steere told the *Ledger*, "I'm not on both sides of the fence. We have no evidence that in vaccinated subjects the gene leads to difficulty. But we recognize the limitations of a study to pick up a rare side effect. It remains a theoretical consideration."

It was reported in the *New York Times* that "Steere had expressed concerns as early as 1995, shortly after the start of the clinical trials, when he said some patients were already getting joint pain and arthritis following vaccination. 'A small percentage of patients have developed joint pain and arthritis following vaccination,' he wrote in a letter to the National Institutes of Health." The *Times* added that "Dr. Steere . . . had told the committee [the FDA's Advisory

Committee] that it was hypothetically possible that the vaccine could set off an autoimmune reaction in which the body's immune system attacks its own tissue, and that this could cause treatment-resistant arthritis."[8]

The article also said, "Even though the Vaccine Advisory Committee recommended approval of Lymerix, the panel's chairwoman, Dr. Patricia L. Ferreiri of the University of Minnesota Medical School, said it had taken the action with unusual ambivalence because of concerns about the possibility of severe reactions." Ultimately the vaccine was approved unanimously and concerns were deemed "theoretical." The *Times* went on to say, "Lymerix is the only clinically proven vaccine to protect against Lyme disease and both the FDA Advisory Committee and the FDA Office of Vaccines have determined that the vaccine is safe."

As well, the *New York Times* reported on concerns expressed by physicians after the vaccine was introduced. A New Jersey rheumatologist said she had told the agency [the FDA] that "21 patients developed severe arthritis soon after being given the vaccine by other doctors," and that she believed the problems were not always linked to [associated with] the vaccine because the vaccine took effect only after three immunizations over the course of a year. Another New Jersey physician reported that 50 of her patients had developed autoimmune arthritis after receiving the vaccine from other doctors, and 30 others appeared to have flare-ups of previous Lyme infections.

Ronald Schell of the University of Wisconsin School of Medicine had documented severe destructive arthritis in hamsters that were given the vaccine and presented his findings at the twelfth annual Conference on Lyme Disease and Other Tick-Borne Disorders (1999) in New York. Doubts about its safety were expressed during the trials and clinical symptoms appeared at that time. Doubts continued after its introduction to the public. Even as complaints came in, and as late as January 2002, the CDC said, "We found no unexpected pattern of adverse events compared to the results of the clinical trial that was done before FDA approval."[9]

THE FOOD AND DRUG ADMINISTRATION
HOLDS HEARINGS ON VACCINE SAFETY

The Food and Drug Administration Advisory Committee consists of a group of physicians and researchers who review data from clinical trials and give recommendations on which vaccines the FDA should approve. It also reviews problems reported to the FDA and sends reports to the Vaccine Adverse Event Reporting System (VAERS). The VAERS is the national safety surveillance program cosponsored by the FDA and CDC. Reports come from individuals, patients, parents, family members, and health care providers. As would be expected, many physicians and those who took the vaccine were unaware of the cause of symptoms, or where to report adverse reactions. They were unsure of the cause of problems or did not choose to file a report.

Two hearings were held in response to reported problems. On November 28, 2001, the Lyme Disease Foundation met with the FDA's vaccine advisory committee, and on January 31, 2002, the Lyme Disease Association met with the committee, demanding answers to a series of questions. Both national organizations fund Lyme disease research, educate the public, and bring information to public forums on behalf of Lyme victims. During these meetings with the FDA, patients, physicians, and scientists told of long-term pain and disability as a result of taking the vaccine.

These are four illustrative cases to show that if you did have an adverse reaction it was long-lasting and no small matter. And it could happen after only one shot.

- A woman took her first dose in May 1999 and experienced flu-like symptoms immediately, but was told her reaction was common. After her second injection her elbows began to ache, with pain spreading down her arms and throughout her body until by November she could barely clasp a carton of milk. She was diagnosed with chronic fatigue, depression, and fibromyalgia, and her doctors eventually suggested that her inflamed joints, aching muscles, and pain might be related to job stress. She learned from news media about a lawsuit and discovered that her problems were indeed the problems of others who had been vaccinated.

- Although too ill to attend the vaccine advisory meeting, a second woman wrote the FDA, "I was given an injection at 4:15 p.m. on 3/15/99 and developed chills, sweats and body aches with a 103.5 degree temperature." She experienced shaking, pounding heart, chattering teeth and now has arthritis that does not go away. She is told that it is permanent.

- Another person's story: "We had moved up from Maryland. We bought some land and a house in the country. We spend a lot of time camping and working outside on our property, so when we heard about the vaccine for Lyme disease we thought it would be a good idea. I had just got a new doctor so I got a complete physical. I was in good health and all my tests came back good. In February I received my first Lymerix shot and became sick very quickly. I had constant aches and pains everywhere in my body. When I received my second Lymerix shot I got even sicker. My doctor then sent me to an arthritis specialist, and I was informed I have fibromyalgia. I had repeatedly told my doctor that it was the Lymerix vaccine that had made me sick, and I refused to take the last shot. This year I was told I have arthritis in my neck. Every bone and muscle in my body hurts."

- A Cape Cod woman, unable to attend the FDA hearing wrote, "I was managing my LD (which I was unaware I had) until the study shots began. Little lumps formed on my knee caps and dark, patchy rashes were visible on the inside of both knees." She describes "brain fog," slurred speech, heightened sensitivity to light and sound, dizziness, headaches, and balance problems. She spoke of her three children, all diagnosed with chronic Lyme disease. "If I were not directly aware of both sides of the vaccine issues I would likely have had all my children vaccinated with Lymerix. Thank goodness, this will not be so."

Among others who spoke was Kathleen Dickson, a biochemist and member of Action/Lyme in Connecticut. Testifying extensively at the January 2002 FDA meeting in Bethesda, Maryland, she stated, "Normal is not less than 'five bands' [of the Western blot]. If the patient has clinical signs of Lyme plus two specific antibody bands, no honest diagnostician would assert that the patient does not have Lyme disease." She emphasized that "normal" is no bands, and no clinical symptoms of Lyme disease.

THE VACCINE MIGHT HAVE BEEN SAFE IF . . .

- You did not have the genetic marker for autoimmune arthritis. When those with HLA-DR4 were injected with the Borrelia burgdorferi protein, there was a possible autoimmune response. The vaccine's purpose was to elicit the production of antibodies against the spirochete to produce an immunity response. With the presence of the genetic marker HLA-DR4, the immune response was exaggerated and the body began attacking its own tissues, as occurs in rheumatoid arthritis.

- You were certain that you had never had Lyme disease. With disagreement over the disease and without a reliable test, it can be hard to know. Injecting the spirochete protein could exacerbate symptoms. Those with Lyme infections may or may not have signs of the disease. Some may have had chronic fatigue or other conditions that were not recognized as Lyme.

- You were sure you carried no current Lyme infection. With an uncertain disease status, the risk of serious side effects from Lyme vaccination increase, as determined by clinical experience and common sense. The cause was associated with a possible autoimmune response. Some who had experienced Lyme in the past mistakenly thought it important to get preventive shots.

- You would not be exposed to tick bites until after the third dose of the vaccine had been given. Shots did not give current protection. Three doses given over the course of a year were required to obtain the degree of immunity described by the researchers. During that year precautions had to be taken as though no injections had been given. In fact, the same precautions had to be taken, whatever the number of shots given, because, even after three doses, the effect was known to decline rapidly.

Those who took the vaccine were not safe from Lyme disease.

THE LYMERIX VACCINE IS PULLED FROM THE MARKET

By February 2002, immediately after the FDA hearings with the Lyme disease organizations, and just two years after its introduction, the Lymerix vaccine was gone, pulled from the market by GlaxoSmithKline because, the company said, it didn't sell. Not mentioned were the chronic illnesses reported to the FDA and the lawsuits against the company, or the negative press that alerted the public and their physicians to the plight of some who took the vaccine.

Ramona DuBose, a spokeswoman for Glaxo said, "Hundreds of thousands were vaccinated [in the first year]. The projections for this year had decreased to 10,000. That's not enough to sustain the product." She said the company did not know why the vaccine did not succeed. Part of it she surmised was the difficulty of asking an otherwise healthy adult to get a series of shots against a potential disease. She added that the company would continue to defend the safety of Lymerix against lawsuits.[10]

The last people to receive the vaccine were those in schools and clinics where supplies were still on hand, and personnel there were as yet unaware that the vaccine had been withdrawn.

CHAPTER THIRTEEN

PREVENTING LYME DISEASE

WHAT TO DO AFTER A TICK BITE—
IT'S MORE THAN TUCKING YOUR
PANTS INTO YOUR SOCKS

We've moved out of the city into a house in the suburbs. We find deer ticks on our dog. We have a three-year old daughter who wants to play outdoors in the yard, and we want her to be able to do that safely. We're thinking about what we can do without constantly checking for ticks. It seems as though part of the solution may be to build a very large deck.

—NEW HOMEOWNER IN NEW JERSEY

Thomas Mather, a professor of entomology at the University of Rhode Island, is among the foremost authorities on preventing tick bites. "Almost everybody knows someone who had Lyme disease," he said in a news article. "[But] we can't even get people to tuck their pants into their socks. They think you can put on a little Deet on your arms and neck and call it a day."[1]

Protection requires more than the traditional reminders to do frequent tick checks. This chapter gives information on how to avoid exposure to ticks, ways to reduce their numbers in your yard, and what to do after you have been outdoors in an environment that could contain ticks. It tells you what to do if you are bitten by a tick, including talking to your doctor about taking a preventive antibiotic. In addition, to reinforce the importance of prevention, I include the latest efforts that have been made by those who would limit antibiotics for Lyme disease and the current status of the Lyme disease problem.

Chapter 3 describes the characteristics of the deer tick and the Borrelia burgdorferi spirochete than can make you vulnerable to Lyme. Dogs are checked and treated promptly, whereas medical care for humans remains uncertain. Chapter 7 points out that we have few doctors willing and knowledgeable enough to treat the disease beyond its early stage. Since thereafter it often becomes ignored or misdiagnosed, avoiding tick bites must become a priority. Taking precautions is far easier than finding the medical care you may need.

LATEST DEVELOPMENTS

The politics of the disease do not go away. With all that we know, and have observed thousands of times, the successes in treating chronic Lyme are often deemed "anecdotal," meaning informal accounts or observations that are not based on documented evidence. Or the diagnosis is denied with the words, "He probably never had the disease in the first place." The science on the persistence of the spirochete, which includes its motility and ability to evade the immune system and antibiotics, and its effects on the body are ignored. With nonsubstantive arguments and attacks on doctors extending far beyond normal professional disagreements, the need to deny chronic Lyme appears more intense than ever.

Assaults on treatment continue to originate from the same small group of physicians who took control of the illness in 1993. It includes Allen Steere, the pioneer in Lyme disease, who is also the physician against whom seventy-five complaints of negligence were filed with the Massachusetts Board of Registration in Medicine in 2000. But, as the public learns the story and more physicians treat the disease as is often necessary, ignoring the signs and risks becomes less possible.

DURING THE FALL OF 2007

Three bills were filed with the Massachusetts state legislature. The purpose was (1) to protect and ensure medical care for Lyme disease and (2) to assure that physicians can make treatment decisions for their patients based on clinical assessment and medical judgment. During this time, another article was published critiquing the Klempner studies of 2000 that denied benefit from continued antibiotics for those with persisting Lyme symptoms.

To protect their position, those on the overtreated side of the controversy took their own actions during the fall of 2007:

- The *New England Journal of Medicine* published an article denying the occurrence of long-term Lyme disease and opposing treatment beyond the guidelines published by the Infectious Diseases Society of America.
- The president of the IDSA wrote a position statement in its journal defending the IDSA Lyme disease committee's restrictive guidelines.
- The Connecticut medical board, with an IDSA physician as expert witness, prepared final arguments in its more than two-year-long case against Charles Ray Jones, the foremost pediatric Lyme specialist in the country who has treated seriously ill children successfully for more than twenty years.

At the same time, Lyme patients in Connecticut held a rally requesting that Henry Feder, Jr. of the University of Connecticut show a test that proves the spirochete has been eradicated. They noted that papers published by the same people who oppose treatment have demonstrated survival of the spirochete. Dr. Feder was the lead author in the just-published *New England Journal of Medicine* article.

THE *NEW ENGLAND JOURNAL OF MEDICINE* ARTICLE

Authors of this article are the same longtime adherents of the over-diagnosed, overtreated theory of the disease, and include Henry Feder, Jr., Eugene Shapiro, Allen Steere, and Gary Wormser. Since 1993 all have promoted the unchanging message in professional journals and in the media. Also included in the author list is "Ad Hoc International Lyme Disease Group." This is not the International Lyme and Associated Tick-Borne Diseases Society that advocates for improved diagnostic criteria and better treatment for persisting disease.

In the article, authors talk of late versus chronic disease, and they assign arbitrary categories for a disease they do not believe can be chronic. For example, those in "category 2" are described as patients who "may or may not have a history of Lyme disease. They have received either a misdiagnosis or diagnosis such as multiple sclerosis that they are unable to accept." Those in

> category 3 disease do not have a history of objective clinical findings that are consistent with Lyme disease, but their serum samples contain antibodies against B. burgdorferi . . . Patients with disease in this category have at most only equivocal evidence of B. burgdorferi infection . . . Although some clinicians would offer patients with category 3 disease an empirical trial of 2 to 4 weeks of an oral antibiotic, such patients should be told that the diagnosis is uncertain and that a benefit from treatment is unlikely.

With this recommendation, patients are asked to take an unnecessary risk for a reason that is questionable at best.

Those designated with "category 4 disease have symptoms associated with post-Lyme disease syndrome." Acknowledged in the article is the cyst form of disease but its possible meaning in terms of treatment is discounted. As described in Chapter 11 on Lyme disease research, the theme of "post-Lyme syndrome" continues.

Included in the article as a supplement is a section, "Advice to Clinicians," saying,

> If there is a diagnosis for which a specific treatment cannot be made, the goal should be to provide emotional support and management of pain, fatigue, or other symptoms as required. Explaining that there is no medication, such as an antibiotic, to cure the condition is one of the most difficult aspects of caring for such patients. Nevertheless, failure to do so in clear and sympathetic language leaves the patient susceptible to unproven and potentially dangerous therapies.[2]

No second opinions for patients are suggested by the authors despite the described complexities of this disease. In fact, patients are discouraged from seeking them.

FROM THE PRESIDENT: THE IDSA STANDS UP FOR LYME DISEASE GUIDELINES

As noted in Chapter 1, Attorney General Richard Blumenthal of Connecticut responded to the IDSA's Lyme guidelines by initiating an investigation into sources that were used by the committee for making its 2006 recommendations. The IDSA president's statement says,

> The Connecticut Attorney General has notified IDSA that he is investigating possible antitrust violations (by not including research that does not support its conclusions) in connection with our 2000 and 2006 Lyme disease guidelines. This unprecedented move against a professional society and its practice guidelines appears to have been initiated on behalf of health care professionals and patient

care advocates who disagree with IDSA recommendations. These individuals maintain that Lyme disease exists in a chronic form.

While saying that nothing replaces the clinician's judgment, the IDSA statement continues:

> We are immensely sympathetic to frustrated patients who have diverse symptoms and who are frustrated that we cannot identify a cause for their symptoms. However, our Society is committed to management recommendations that rely on data, interpreted by experienced clinicians and researchers, to formulate recommendations for what approaches are effective and safe.[3]

New ILADS Article Supports Treatment for Lyme Disease

During the fall of 2007, an article was published, authored by Raphael Stricker of the International Lyme and Associated Tick-Borne Diseases Society, and Lorraine Johnson, executive director of the California Lyme Disease Association. It notes once again that the Klempner studies of 2000, discussed in Chapter 11, were short-term, three-month studies using low-dose treatments. A group of patients who had Lyme disease in the past with persisting symptoms were treated by regimens that included oral doxycycline and thirty days of intravenous ceftriaxone. These were the studies that concluded there was no benefit from continued treatment for ongoing Lyme symptoms.

Among the points made in the Stricker and Johnson article was one that Andrea Gaito and Daniel Cameron had made earlier in 2004.[4] Patients in the Klempner study had already been sick for an average of 4.7 years and treated with an average of three courses of antibiotics. Therefore, the 2000 Klempner studies were, in effect, re-treatment studies for patients who had already failed earlier treatment. It was "too little too late."[5]

Also, in the fall of 2007, Brian Fallon's study at Columbia University's Department of Psychiatry was published. It was a randomized, placebo-controlled trial of intravenous antibiotic therapy on Lyme encephalopathy.[6] The effect of repeated intravenous therapy for neurological Lyme disease showed cognitive improvement after a period of twelve weeks, and that relapse might occur when the treatment was discontinued.

Ticks are Hardy and Difficult to Detect

There are a number of ways to reduce your chances of getting bitten. Some are more obvious and well known than others. The immature nymph is no larger than the size of a period at the end of a sentence, with an adult tick the size of a poppy seed. Whether nymphs or adults, deer ticks are difficult to detect, and both transmit Lyme disease.

They are hardy and live in a wide range of climate conditions. They survive winter temperatures and become active whenever the temperature rises above 35 to 40 degrees Fahrenheit. They are found in low-lying vegetation, not in overhanging tree branches, and are attracted by body warmth and the exhaled carbon dioxide of animals and humans. They do not drop from trees.

Although "tick season" is considered late spring and summer, tick bites occur in almost every month of the year. There is no "safe" season.

What You Can Do to Protect Against Tick Bites

The following guidelines come from federal, state, and local governments, the U.S. Department of Agriculture, Lyme disease organizations, and from personal experiences.

- Recommended are long pants tucked into socks, shirt tucked into waistband, long sleeves, and hat. Since, however, ticks hide in collars and folds of clothes, clothing should be removed and examined closely after exposure to tick habitats.

- To make ticks more visible, wear light-colored clothes, socks, and shoes.
- Ticks may be more easily seen on bare skin than on clothes. Skin must be examined frequently, even every two or three hours, while you are outdoors to discover any tick attachment. Even though you are clothed, so it takes it more time, a tick will find skin. It will crawl onto you and then move upward to a waistband or neck until it finds a place to attach.
- Clothes worn in the outdoors should be put into the dryer for at least twenty minutes, probably a half hour, at high heat. Some say more. Ticks are most vulnerable to dehydration. Sometimes, if the water temperature is not high enough, they survive the washing machine.
- Ticks are difficult to see in hair, on the hairline, behind the knees and ears. They prefer inaccessible places such as the groin or under the arms. Safest, after yard work, or exposure to fields and woods, is a shower and shampoo. However, showers will remove only ticks that have not yet attached.
- All shoes should be carefully examined, or left outside the door after being outdoors. Examine them again before putting them back on.

Parents with experience in serious Lyme disease have said, "I don't want my children outside in fields and woods long enough for a tick to attach. I want them inside at least very three or four hours to check their socks and clothing. I don't want to give ticks a chance to attach to their skin. We leave our shoes outdoors, and drop our clothes into a plastic bag and into the washing machine. Jackets go into the dryer. We check our small children's skin and hair, and have the older ones check themselves. We give the children baths and take showers. We don't take chances."

AVOIDING TICK EXPOSURE

The Massachusetts Department of Public Health recommends that Deet (N, N—diethyl-m-toluamide) products such as BUG OUT, CUTTER, OFF!, Off! Skintastic, Skintastic for Kids, 3M Ultrathon, or a similar product be sprayed on outer clothing and exposed skin, but not the face. Do not overapply or saturate clothing. At a maximum, the concentration should never exceed 35 percent, 15 percent for children. Deet is a repellent that does not kill ticks unless they are in direct contact with the solution. It may be sprayed on the back of the neck, but not on the face, which should be protected by hats and by checking for ticks.

Permethrin, a pesticide that acts as a neurotoxin, is another chemical used for preventing tick bites. It is an insecticide that is applied only to clothing, not skin, and lasts through several washings. These chemicals, Deet and permethrin, are useful for field trips and other occasions, but not everyone is comfortable using either of them on a regular basis, and they do not eliminate the need for vigilance.

TICK CONTROL

Ticks have no natural enemies with the possible exception of guinea hens, who eat ticks and other bugs. Although having guinea hens is impractical for most people, they have been found effective in tick control. They require several acres of more or less open land and are too noisy for residential areas. If penned for the first week or so, they can be let out and will remain on the property.

Other methods of tick control include using Damminex tubes containing permethrin. The U.S. Environmental Protection Agency classifies it as a carcinogen, and it is toxic to honeybees, aquatic insects, shrimp, and other organisms. Biodegradable Damminex tubes, containing cotton treated with permethrin, may be used in the yard. Mice bring the cotton back to their nests where ticks that are present may be killed.

Dandux 4-Poster deer treatment bait and feed stations have been set up in some park areas. A control bin contains whole kernel corn. There are two entrances to the bins. They are refilled as needed. When the deer feed from the bins, their heads and necks are exposed to rollers containing a pesticide, which kills the ticks.

High fences, with eight feet recommended, have been used around property, and longer hunting seasons have been tried to reduce the deer populations. But, whatever else is done, mice populations continue to thrive and individual precautions are required to prevent tick exposure.

REDUCING THE NUMBER OF TICKS IN YOUR YARD

Ticks prefer shaded, protected, moist locations where they can better avoid dehydration. They like the dampness of seaside air and reside in grassy areas near the ocean. They are less likely to be found in sunny lawns, but you can't be sure. Park benches have been found to offer protection for ticks seeking a blood meal from animals or humans. Recommendations for limiting ticks in your environment come from health departments, park services, and Lyme disease organizations.

- Keep grass cut and shrubs trimmed.
- Remove brush and leaf piles, which are favorite locations for ticks.
- Woodpiles are likely to contain ticks. Keep them away from play areas.
- Use wood chips around outdoor recreation areas and as a barrier between yard and woods.
- Avoid sitting on tree stumps, wooden park benches, and stone walls. Ticks like damp crevices and protected locations.
- Walk on woodland trails that are at least six feet wide.
- Be careful when walking through shore beach grass which often contains ticks that attach to your legs.
- Be aware that kneeling amid foliage while gardening exposes your head and neck to ticks.
- Remember that pets may bring ticks into your home.

Even after being careful, if you find a deer tick on the skin and you can brush it off, there is no need to worry. Says a summer resident of Nantucket, "I play tennis and the court is surrounded by scrubby tick-filled bushes and lots of wind. Occasionally, a tick blows onto the court. When I'm through playing, I use a brush in case I miss something on the back of my legs."

What to Do If You Are Bitten by a Tick

If, despite precautions, you find a tick that is already attached to your skin, you must first remove it. You will then have to consider what you wish to do next. Without knowing whether or not it is infected with Lyme or other tick-borne diseases, or how much saliva it has introduced into your body, most people will take the next step of opting for a preventive antibiotic.

- If you find a tick that you cannot brush off, use fine-tipped tweezers pressed into the skin around the head and pull gently straight, at a right angle to the skin (see Chapter 3). Only the head section is attached. The rest of the tick remains outside your body. If you pull only on the body, the head will remain inside where the saliva can cause infection.
- If you cannot or do not want to do this yourself, or don't have access to tweezers, don't try to dig it out or use alcohol, Vaseline, nail polish, or a match. People have used these methods in the past, but they don't work and may cause the tick to burrow deeper, and may increase your chance of infection. Go to your doctor or emergency room. If the tick comes off, place it in a bag and save it for the doctor.
- You can't assume you know how long the tick was attached. If you had known it was attached, you would have already removed it. The longer it is there, the greater the risk of contracting Lyme.
- Save the tick in a sealed plastic bag. Do not place it in alcohol or it cannot be tested. It has a hard shell and will not disintegrate.

You may be asked later if you are sure it was a deer tick. If a facility such as a state or university testing laboratory is available, you might have the tick tested to find out whether it carried the spirochete.

- Request at least a week of preventive doxycycline from your doctor. If you could be or are pregnant, or in the case of a young child, another antibiotic, not in the tetracycline family, will be substituted as suggested in the ILADS treatment guidelines.

There is no reason for you to take the risk that the tick is not infected with Lyme or other tick-borne diseases. Without knowing the status of the tick, and especially in a highly endemic area, I would want two or four weeks of preventive medicine. We have no definitive answer as to how long the antibiotic needs to be taken, and you should have input into the amount of risk you are willing to accept.

Talk to your doctor about your possible exposure to the tick and let the doctor know if you prefer the conservative approach in order to minimize your chances of contracting a Lyme infection. If a pink or reddish area develops around the bite, or has already formed—and it doesn't have to be a bull's-eye rash—I would not accept "local irritation" as the cause. I would want several weeks of antibiotic, perhaps with a higher-than-standard dose just to be sure. The following recommendations summarize information given in Chapter 8 on treating the disease.

- If I had possible exposure to ticks and noted an unexplained rash that fitted the description of Lyme rash but the tick was no longer present, I would not accept "possible spider bite" as the reason. I would want the preventive antibiotic.
- If I had spent time outdoors in conditions that could have exposed me to ticks, and I experienced unexplained symptoms, I would consider the possibility of a Lyme infection and would ask for evaluation. With malaise, fatigue, and light-headedness

that did not go away in a few days, I would want a preventive antibiotic. Just because I didn't see the tick, I would not take a chance that what I had "could be a virus." It could be Lyme.

- If I had been ill for months and years with misdiagnoses or undiagnosed disease, such as chronic fatigue syndrome, fibromyalgia, or more serious illnesses, I would seek evaluation by a Lyme-literate physician who treats chronic Lyme disease.
- If I were in a job or activity that included regular exposure to ticks, I would consider keeping a bottle of doxycycline on hand in my medicine cabinet. (This requires a prescription from your family doctor.)

In most cases after removing the tick and taking the preventive antibiotic, you can expect no more problems. If you become ill, you will have to take further steps to ensure adequate treatment.

IF YOU HAVE LYME SYMPTOMS AND HAVE TAKEN A PREVENTIVE ANTIBIOTIC . . .

You can't assume that the problem will go away. Your aching body and unusual, persisting fatigue that are not relieved by a night's sleep may not be due to long hours at work or cleaning out the basement.

- Ask for a refill, or two, of your prescription and consider increasing the dose or changing the antibiotic. Discuss with your doctor at the outset your desire to avoid unnecessary risk.
- The refill will likely be given. If it is not, and your doctor expresses doubt that you have the disease, telling you that a few weeks of antibiotics are enough, say that you are aware of the controversy, and that you want to be assured of protection against this disease. You want to minimize your risk. Bring information that supports your request, such as articles that validate the possible need for continuing treatment, or this book. When I called for a refill and didn't get it, I went to my doctor's office

and waited to see him. I said I didn't want to take a chance on getting Lyme. I was given two refills.

- If you are told that your condition could be something other than Lyme, be willing to accept further tests that might indicate that you have acquired another illness. If the diagnosis is unavailable or becomes chronic fatigue, or pain for which there is no test, be aware that this is what commonly occurs when Lyme is not diagnosed correctly.
- If you continue to be ill, take a Western blot Lyme test, knowing that it is not diagnostic and doesn't influence your decision. You want the result of it in your record to compare with possible future laboratory tests.
- Monitor your symptoms (see appendix for list of possible symptoms) and keep notes.
- If you are left untreated, seek another physician for continuing antibiotics. If, in your view, medical care remains inadequate, contact the Lyme disease organizations, including the International Lyme and Associated Tick-Borne Diseases Society.

In these pages I've told you about the disease, how it was discovered, and how it relates to our experience with other infectious diseases. At the time of its discovery a period of years was required to connect the rash, the joint symptoms, the tick vector, and the bacteria that it carries. The possible neurological symptoms have only recently been included in the criteria that were developed by the Council of State and Territorial Epidemiologists for use in reporting the disease, and that are used in the federal government's case definition of the disease.

The controversy on Lyme leaves the public with two medical camps on treating the disease, each almost diametrically opposed to the other. The differences leave physicians unprepared to treat Lyme disease that is not caught early. Because of the politics, confrontation with insurance companies is often required for reimbursement of the costs of the illness, necessitating many phone calls and letters and the keeping of much documentation and many records. Schools have children in their classrooms who are fatigued and unable to learn because of un-recognized or misdiagnosed Lyme.

Guidelines that were issued by a private organization, The Infectious Diseases Society of America, act to restrict progress and limit treatment as occurs with no other disease. Not everyone can expect to recover completely from long-neglected illness, but all can, and should, seek the best medical care available for a disease that can enter joints, brains, and hearts. Lest others fall into the same net that I did, I've written this book to give information that helped me and others climb out of an abyss.

It is an outrage that so many are dismissed by the medical profession to languish out of public view with unevaluated and misdiagnosed ill-ness. As found by Lyme-literate physicians, at least 10 percent of those who get Lyme disease are becoming chronically ill, and the cause relates to lack of treatment. Many are on antidepressants, pain-killers, and steroids. It is their good fortune if the misdiagnosis is no more than "chronic fatigue syndrome." For many others, the misdiagnosis can be multiple sclerosis, or worse. If ongoing or recurring Lyme happens to be recognized, but doesn't go away promptly, people are told that "it can't be Lyme," or "studies say that continued antibiotics are of no benefit."

All the while, physicians from the two camps argue about who is right and who is wrong. All attempts to effect a reasoned solution have so far failed. The theme of "post-Lyme syndrome," or post-Lyme arthritis, continues to be played without a shred of hard sci-ence. The public is caught in the middle, exposed to information that long ago was found to be wrong, and trying to stay safe from a disease that is present right outside their windows.

The war on doctors is so intense that those who treat persisting Lyme regularly face investigation and possible loss of their medical li-censes by IDSA-dominated state boards. Needless to say, treatment for this common disease is scarce. Physician clinical judgment has lost ground for Lyme far more than it has for other conditions. But when enough of the public becomes aware, the current situation can change.

APPENDIX:
SYMPTOM CHECKLIST

The following are possible indicators of Lyme. You may have one or more symptoms, but having them does not diagnose Lyme. However, the list helps those who may have been exposed to the disease to consider what they are experiencing. Symptoms can then be brought to physicians for evaluation of the illness.

1. Unexplained fevers, sweats, chills, or flushing
2. Unexplained weight change—loss or gain
3. Fatigue, tiredness, poor stamina
4. Unexplained hair loss
5. Swollen glands: list areas
6. Sore throat
7. Testicular/pelvic pain
8. Unexplained menstrual irregularity
9. Unexplained milk production, breast pain
10. Irritable bladder or bladder dysfunction
11. Sexual dysfunction or loss of libido
12. Upset stomach
13. Change in bowel function—constipation or diarrhea
14. Chest pain or rib soreness
15. Shortness of breath, cough

16. Heart palpitations, pulse skips, heart bloc
17. Any history of a heart murmur or valve prolapse
18. Joint pain or swelling: list joint
19. Stiffness of joints, neck, or back
20. Muscle pain or cramps
21. Twitching of the face or other muscles
22. Headache
23. Neck creeks and cracks, neck stiffness, neck pain
24. Tingling, numbness, burning, or stabbing sensations
25. Facial paralysis (Bell's palsy)
26. Eyes/vision: double, blurry, floaters, increased light sensitivity
27. Ears: buzzing, ringing, ear pain, sound sensitivity
28. Increased motion sickness, vertigo, poor balance
29. Lightheadedness, wooziness
30. Tremor
31. Confusion, difficulty in thinking
32. Difficulty with concentration, reading
33. Forgetfulness, poor short-term memory
34. Disorientation: getting lost; going to wrong places
35. Difficulty with speech or writing
36. Mood swings: irritability, depression
37. Disturbed sleep—too much, too little, early awakening
38. Exaggerated symptoms or worse hangover from alcohol

(Source: International Lyme and Associated Diseases Guidelines, 2002, Joseph Burrascano, M.D., www.Lymenet.org).

RESOURCES

The following addresses, websites, and telephone numbers are useful sources of information on support groups, physicans who treat Lyme disease, and other help, such as pamphlets and videos. These organizations are located in various parts of the country and Canada, and are listed alphabetically.

California Lyme Disease Association

Phyllis Mervine, President
P.O. Box 707
Weaverville, California 06093
tel. 310-456-3625
www.LymeDisease.org

Publisher of *The Lyme Times*

Canadian Lyme Disease Foundation

Jim Wilson, President
Westbank, British Columbia
jimwilson@telus.net
tel. 1-250-768-0978
www.canalyme.com

Resources

Empire (New York) State Lyme Disease Association
Eva Haugh, President
P.O. Box 874
Manorville, New York, 11949
eva@EmpireStateLDA.org
www.empirestatelymediseaseassociation

Greater Hartford Support and Action Group
Randy Sykes
model1918@sbcglobal.net
1-860-658-9938
www.CTLymedisease.org

International Lyme and Associated Diseases Society
P.O. Box 34161
Bethesda, Maryland 20827
tel. 301-263-1080
lymedocs@aol.org
www.ILADS.org

Iowa Lyme Disease Group
mstarfraj@cloudburst9.net

Lyme Education Awareness Program
P.O. Box 2654
Mesa, Arizona 85214
tel. 1-480-219-6869
tinajgarcia@yahoo.com

Lyme Disease Association
President, Patricia V. Smith
P.O. Box 1438
Jackson, New Jersey 08527
1-888-366-6611
www.LymeDiseaseAssociation.org

Lyme Disease Association of Cape Cod, Chapter of Lyme Disease Association

P.O. Box 304

West Barnstable, Massachusetts 02668

LDAofCC@aol.com

Lyme Disease Association of Southeastern Pennsylvania

P.O. Box 181

Pocopson, Pennsylvania 19366

Lyepa@Lymepa.org

tel. 1-610-388-7333

Lyme Disease Association, Rhode Island Chapter of Lyme Disease Association

jumerol@yahoo.com

Lyme Disease Foundation

Karen Forschner, founder

P.O. Box 352

Tolland, Connecticut 06094

tel. 1-860-870-0070

info@lyme.org

founded in 1988 as the first Lyme organization

Lyme Disease Network of Middle Tennessee

lyme@tnlyme.org

Lyme Disease Network of South Carolina

P.O. Box 6634

Columbia, South Carolina 29260

tel. 1-803-798-5963

Lyme@sc-lyme.org

Massachusetts Lyme Disease Awareness Association

John Coughlan, President

P.O. Box 1916

Mashpee, Massachusetts 02649
1-508-564-7445

Massachusetts
Kay Lyon
b1og7@verizon.net
www.Lymesite.com
Mimi Winer 1-508-653-5569

Michigan Lyme Disease Association
Linda Lobes, Founder and President
1-888-784-5963

publishes monthly newsletter *Tick Tock*
membership address: 35431 Brush Street, Wayne, Michigan 48184

Minnesota Lyme Fighters Advocacy
Tracie Schissel
1-218-829-5963
Leslie Wermers
1-952-217-5946
www.lymefighers.org

National Capital Lyme and Tick-Borne Diseases Association
P.O. Box 8211
McLean, Virginia 22106
tel. 1-703-821-8833
natcaplyme@natcaplyme.org
www.natcaplyme.org

National Research Fund for Tick-Borne Diseases
P.O. Box 643
Wilton, Connecticut 06897
Leo Shea III, Ph.D., neurologist
1-917-439-3061
www.nrftd.org

Ohio

w.w.w.geocities.com/ldbullseye

Oregon Lyme Disease Network

tel. 1-541-312-3081

lyme@junipermeadow.com

Ridgefield Lyme Disease Task Force

66 Prospect Street

Ridgefield, Connecticut

RLDF@comcast.net

tel. 1-203-431-7006

Texas Lyme Disease Association

P.O. Box 1811

Colleyville, Texas 76034

The Lanford Foundation—Lifelyme, inc.

Sandi Lanford, founder

13039 Gopher Wood Trail

Tallahassee, Florida 32312

1-850-906-9108

www.Lifelyme@yahoo.org

Time for Lyme, Inc.

P.O. Box 31269

Greenwich, Connecticut 06831

timeforlyme@aol.com

Turn the Corner Foundation, Inc.

15 West 63rd St. suite 23A

New York, NY 10023

tel. 1-212-580-6262

info@turnthecorner.org

Resources

Washington State Lyme Disease Association
information and support groups
www.walyme.org

BOOKS

Polly Murray, *The Widening Circle: A Lyme Disease Pioneer Tells Her Story,* St. Martin's Press, New York, 1996

Karen Forschner, *Everything You Need to Know About Lyme Disease and Other Disorders,* John Wiley, 2nd edition, 2003

Denise Lang with Kenneth Liegner, *Coping with Lyme Disease: A Practical Guide For Dealing with Diagnosis and Treatment,* Henry Holt, 3rd edition, New York, 2003

Jonathan Edlow, *Bull's Eye, Unraveling the Mystery of Lyme Disease,* Yale University Press, New Haven, Connecticut, 2003

Karen P. Yerges and Rita Stanley, *Confronting Lyme: What Patient Stories Teach Us,* Mitre's Touch Gallery, 1414 Adams Avenue, La Grande, Oregon, 97850, 2005

Sue Vogan, *No Compassion Observed,* BioMed Publishing Group, South Lake Tahoe, California, 2007

Joseph J. Burrascano, Jr., M.D., *Diagnostic Hints and Treatment Guidelines for Lyme and Other Tick-Borne Diseases,* available at website of the International Lyme and Associated Tick-Borne Diseases Society (ILADS) at ILADS.org

Expert Review of Anti-Infective Therapy, Evidence-Based Guidelines for the Management of Lyme Disease, The International Lyme and Associated Diseases Society, P.O. Box 341461, Bethesda, Maryland 20827 Also published in the National Guidelines Clearing House, www.guideline.gov

Notes

Chapter 2

1. David Whelan, "Lyme, Inc." *Forbes Magazine*, March 12, 2007.

2. Lady Mary Wortley Montagu, *Letters of the Right Honourable Lady M—y W—y M—e: Written During her Travels in Europe, Asia and Africa . . .*, vol. 1 (Aix: Anthony Henricy, 1796), pp. 167–169. Available online at http:www.fordham.edu/halsall/mod/montagu-smallpox.html.

3. Fleming, Alexander, A. "Fleming on a Remarkable Bacteriolyte Found in Tissues and Secretions," *Proceedings of the Royal Society* 93, ser. B. (1922): 307–317.

4. Mark Jerome Walters, *Six Modern Plagues and How We Are Causing Them,* (Washington, D.C.: Island Press, 2001).

Chapter 3

1. Polly Murray, *The Widening Circle* (N.Y.: St. Martin's Press, 1996).

2. Jonathan Edlow, *Bull's-Eye, Unraveling the Medical Mystery of Lyme Disease* (New Haven: Yale University Press, 2003).

Chapter 4

1. Guidelines from the Infectious Diseases Society of America, Practice Guidelines for the Treatment of Lyme Disease, *Infectious Diseases Society of America Guidelines* (Arlington, Va.: 2006), p. 18.

2. Brian Fallon, "A Controlled Study of Cognitive Deficits in Children," *Journal of Neuropsychiatry* 13. 2001: 500–507.

3. Transcript of the hearing on chronic Lyme disease, Albany, New York, November 27, 2001, p. 258.

4. *Guidelines*, p. 36.

5. Transcript of the Connecticut legislative hearing on chronic Lyme disease, Hartford, January 29, 2004, p. 12.

6. David Grann, "Stalking Dr. Steere over Lyme Disease," *New York Times Magazine,* June 17, 2001.

7. Transcript of the Albany, New York, legislative hearing on chronic Lyme disease, Albany, New York, November 27, 2001, p. 321.

8. Dorothy Wall, *Encounters with the Invisible* (College Station: Texas A&M University Press, 2006).

9. Transcript of the Connecticut hearing, pp. 84–86.

Chapter 5

1. Sam T. Donta, MD, Continuing Education Course, Boston University, 2001.

2. Sam T. Donta, MD, letter to author, January 12, 2007.

3. Ibid.

Chapter 6

1. Jamie Talan, "Experts Are Split over Diagnosis and Treatment of Tick-Borne Illness," Newsday.com, May 22, 2007.

2. http:www.Medscape.com/viewarticle557464.

3. *Boston Globe,* June 25, 2007, p. C4.

4. Jane Gross, "Some Patients Feel Lost," *New York Times,* July 7, 2001.

Chapter 7

1. Editorial, "Doxycycline for Tick Bites—Not for Everyone," *New England Journal of Medicine* Vol. 345, no. 2 (2001): 133–134.

2. Allen Steere, "The Over Diagnosis of Lyme Disease," *Journal of the American Medical Association* 14, no. 269 (1993): 1812–1816.

3. *Lymelight* (The Lyme Disease Foundation, Tolland, Connecticut, newsletter), 2000.

4. David Grann, "Stalking Dr. Steere Over Lyme Disease," *New York Times Magazine,* June 17, 2001, accessed on www.nytimes.com.

5. Michael Lasandra, "Patients to Protest Talk by Lyme Disease Discoverer," *Boston Herald,* November 3, 1999.

6. *Lyme Alliance Newsletter* (Michigan), 2000.

7. Lyme Disease Foundation (Tolland, CT), *Lyme Times,* Winter/Spring 2000.

8. Holcomb Noble, "Questioning Long-Term Lyme Disease," *New York Times,* May 23, 2000, accessed on www.nytimes.com.

9. Holcomb Noble, "Lyme Disease Doctors Rally Behind a Colleague Under Inquiry," *New York Times,* November 10, 2000, accessed on www.nytimes.com.

10. David France, "War Over Lyme Disease," *Newsweek,* November 11, 2000, accessed on www.msnbc.com/news.

11. Stephanie Ramp, "The Dirty Truth Behind Lyme Disease Research," *Fairfield County* (Connecticut) *Weekly,* November 10, 2000, accessed on www.pahealthsystems .com/archive.

12. Stephanie Ramp, *East Hampton* (New York) *Star,* November 16, 2000, accessed on www.easthamptonstar.com.

13. Mark Klempner et al., "Two Controlled Trials of Antibiotic Treatment of Patients with Persistent Symptoms and History of Lyme Disease," *New England Journal of Medicine* 345, no. 2 (2001): 85–92.

14. Gina Kolata, "Lyme Disease Is Hard to Catch and Easy to Treat," *New York Times,* June 13, 2001, accessed on www.nytimes.com.

15. J.D. Heyman, Joanne Fowler, "The Hidden Plague," *People,* June 16, 2003.

16. Edie Clark, "Trouble in Paradise," *Yankee Magazine,* July/August 2007.

17. Michael Lasandra, "Patients to Protest Talk by Lyme Disease Discoverer," *Boston Herald,* November 3, 1999.

Chapter 8

1. Robert Nadelman, "Single Dose Doxycycline for Prevention of Lyme Disease," *New England Journal of Medicine* 345 (2001): 1348–1350.

2. Rebecca Pollard, "The Lyme Enigma," *Bostonia,* 2000, accessed on www.bu.edu/ alumni/bostonia.

3. Sam T. Donta, "Macrolide Therapy of Chronic Lyme Disease," *MedSciMonit,* 2003, 9(11): 136–142.

4. Sam T. Donta, "Tetracycline Therapy for Chronic Lyme Disease," *Clinical Infectious Diseases* 25, suppl. 1 (1997): 852–856.

5. Lesley Ann Fein, "Retrospective Analysis of 160 Patients with Lyme Disease," presented at the nineth annual International Conference on Lyme Borreliosis, April 1996.

6. *Lyme Times,* November/December 1998.

Chapter 9

1. Irwin Vanderhoof et al., "Lyme Disease: The Cost to Society," *Contingencies,* Jan/Feb 1993, pp. 42–48.

2. Mary Carmichael, "The Great Lyme Debate, Patients Ache as Doctors Disagree About Whether There Is a Chronic Form of the Tick-Borne Malady," *Newsweek* August 6, 2007, p. 42.

Chapter 10

1. Lawrence K. Altman, "Annual Exam Gives Bush Good Marks for Health," *New York Times,* August 9, 2007, accessed on www.nytimes.com.

2. Cynthia McCormick, *Cape Cod Times,* August 10, 2007, accessed on www.capecodtimes.com.

3. Christopher Rowland, *Boston Globe,* March 13, 2004.

4. Transcript of the hearing on chronic Lyme disease, Albany, New York, November 27, 2001, p. 227.

Chapter 11

1. Jarma Oksi, "Borrelia burgdorfer Detected by Culture and PCR in Relapse of Lyme Borreliosis," *Annals of Medicine* 35 (1999): 225–232.

2. Kenneth Liegner, letter to the editor, *American Academy of Dermatology* February 28 (1993): 312–314.

3. Edward Masters, "Clinical Differentiation of Lyme Erythma, Migrans, Loxocelism and Cutaneous Anthrax," *Clinical Practice,* no. 3 (1994): 207–208.

4. Reinhard Straubinger, B.A. Summers, V.F. Chang, M.J.G. Appel, "Persistence of Borrelia burgdorferi in Experimentally Infected Dogs," *Journal of Clinical Microbiology* 35, no. 1 (1997): 11–16.

5. Sam T. Donta, "Tetracycline Therapy for Chronic Lyme Disease," *Clinical Infectious Diseases,* 25 suppl. 1 (1997): 852–856.

6. Sam T. Donta, "Late and Chronic Lyme Disease," *Clinics of North America* 86 (2002): 341–349.

7. Sam T. Donta, "The Existence of Chronic Lyme Disease," *Current Treatment Options in Infectious Diseases* 3 (2001): 261–262.

8. Sam T. Donta, "Macrolide Therapy of Chronic Lyme Disease," *Medical Science Monitor* 11 (2003): p. 136–142.

9. Alan Macdonald, "Alzheimer's Neuroborreliosis with Trans-Synaptic Spread of Infection and Neurofibrillary Tangles Derived from Intraneural Spirochetes," *Med Hypotheses,* 68 (4) (2007): 822–826.

10. Sam T. Donta, "Reactivation of Lyme Disease Following OspA Vaccine," *Journal of Antimicrobial Agents* 17 (2001): 16–17.

11. Transcript of the Connecticut legislative hearing on chronic Lyme disease, Hartford, January 29, 2004, p. 21.

12. Ibid., p. 22.

13. Ibid., p. 136.

14. Ibid., p. 147.

15. Editorial, Allen Steere, *New England Journal of Medicine*, 15, no. 7 (1993): 274–275.

16. Robert Schoen, *Connecticut Medicine* 53, no. 6 (1989): 335–337.

17. *Journal of Infectious Diseases* 166, no. 2 (1992): 440–444.

18. E.L. Logian, R.F. Kaplan and A.C. Steere, "Chronic Neurologic Manifestations of Lyme Disease," *New England Journal of Medicine* (1990): 1438–1444.

19. Henry M. Feder, "Differences Are Voiced by Two Lyme Camps at a Connecticut Public Hearing on Insurance Coverage of Lyme Disease," *Pediatrics* 105, no. 4 (2000): 855–857.

20. Mark Klempner et al., "Two Controlled Trials of Antibiotic Treatment in Patients with Persistent Symptoms and a History of Lyme Disease," *New England Journal of Medicine*, 345 (July 12, 2001): pp. 85–92.

21. Gary Wormer et al., "Duration of Antibiotic Therapy for Early Lyme Disease, A Randomized, Double-Blind, Placebo-Controlled Trial, *Annals of Internal Medicine* 138 (2003): 697–704.

22. ILADS Position Paper in response to Wormser Study on Duration of Antibiotic Treatment.

23. Eugene Shapiro, editorial, *New England Journal of Medicine*, July 12, 2001.

24. Robert Nadelman, "Prophylaxis with Single Dose Doxycycline for Prevention of Lyme Disease After an Ixodes Scapularis Tick Bite," *New England Journal of Medicine* 345, no. 2 (2001): 79–84.

25. Nancy Shadick, "Musculoskeletal and Neurologic Outcomes in Patients with Previous Lyme Disease," *Annals of Internal Medicine* 131 (1999): 919–926.

26. Robert Kalish, "Evaluation of Study Patients with Lyme Disease 10–20 Year Follow-Up," *Journal of Infectious Diseases* 183 (2001): 453–460.

Chapter 12

1. Pamela Weintraub, testimony. Transcript of the hearing on chronic Lyme disease, Albany, New York, November 27, 2001, p. 295.

2. Marcia Angell, *The Truth About Drug Companies: How They Deceive Us and What to Do About It* (New York: Random House, 2005).

3. Jim Wilson, AIIC, president of the Canadian Lyme Disease Foundation on behalf of our board of directors, letter to Governor Jon Corzine, August 27, 2007.

4. Sam T. Donta, "Reactivation of Lyme Disease Following Osp A Vaccine," *Journal of Antimicrobial Agents* 17 (2002): 516–517.

Notes

5. Holcomb Noble, "3 Suits Say Lyme Vaccine Caused Severe Arthritis," *New York Times,* June 13, 2000, accessed on www.nytimes.com.

6. Wyatt Olsen, "Women Decry Miseries of Lyme Disease Vaccine," *Asbury Park* (New Jersey) *Press,* August 13, 2000, accessed on www.app.com.

7. Edward Silverman, "Warning Was Dropped on Lyme Vaccination," *Newark* (New Jersey) *Star Ledger*, June 14, 2000, accessed on www.njvoices.com.

8. Holcomb Noble, "Concerns Grow Over Reaction To Lyme Shots," *New York Times*, November 21, 2000, accessed on www.nytimes.com.

9. "CDC Affirms Safety of Lyme Vaccine," *Newsday,* January 18, 2002.

10. *Cape Cod Times*, March 2, 2002, accessed on www.capecodtimes.com.

Chapter 13

1. Andrew Rimas, "He Wants Ticks To Be Taken More Seriously," *Boston Globe,* June 4, 2007.

2. H.M.Feder, Jr., B.J.B. Johnson, S. O'Connell, A.C. Steere, E. Shapiro, G. Wormser, and the ad hoc international Lyme group, "A Critical Appraisal of 'Chronic Lyme Disease,'" *New England Journal of Medicine* 357, no. 14 (2007): 1422–1430.

3. *IDSA News,* Infectious Diseases Society of America, "From the President: IDSA Stands Up For Lyme Disease Guidelines," 17, no. 2 (2007).

4. Daniel Cameron, Andrea Gaito, and Nick Harris, "Evidence-Based Guidelines for the Management of Lyme Disease," *Expert Review of Anti-Infective Therapy* 2, 1 suppl. (2004): S1-S13.

5. Raphael Stricker and Lorraine Johnson, Expert Review of Anti-Infective Therapy, 5, no. 5 (2007): 759–762.

6. Brian Fallon et al., "A Randomized, Placebo-Controlled Trial of Repeated IV Antibiotic Therapy for Lyme Encepalopathy," *Journal of Neurology* (2007): published online before printing, October 10, 2007.

INDEX

Index

Index

Index

Index

About the Authors

Constance A. Bean, author of six previous health-related books, is a graduate of Mount Holyoke College with a Master of Public Health degree from Yale University. She was a staff member at the Massachusetts Institute of Technology for 14 years and a lecturer at Northeastern University for five years. Since 2000, having experienced Lyme, she has researched the disease, spoken with large numbers of people who are ill, attended Lyme disease meetings and conferences, including those of the Massachusetts Department of Public Health Task Force on Lyme and Tick-Borne Diseases, and the Cape Cod and Islands Lyme Disease Task Force.

Constance Bean is among the small group of founders of the natural childbirth movement in this country, and a co-founder of the Boston Association for Childbirth Education, Inc., where she organized and taught parent classes, provided labor support, educated hospital staffs, and worked for change in antiquated hospital policies and regulations. Her book *Methods of Childbirth* became a classic for parents and professionals. She has long been an activist in environmental and health affairs. For the past six years, she has served on her town's board of health. She lives in Wayland, Massachusetts, and on Cape Cod.

Lesley Ann Fein, MD, MPH grew up in South Africa where she received a Bachelor of Science degree with honors. While in South Africa, she was part of a group of students who started a free clinic for indigent farm laborers, which is now integrated into the medical school program in Johannesburg. She then moved to the U.S., where she received her Master of Public Health degree from Columbia University. She received her medical degree (with distinction) from George Washington University in 1981, where she was also accepted into the AOA Honor society, and received an award for academic excellence from the American Medical Women's Association. She completed her internal medicine residency at Mt. Sinai Hospital in New York and completed a Rheumatology fellowship at New York University. When she entered the rheumatology program, she had already identified her interest in the relationship between infections and auto-immune diseases. She spent a year of the NYU fellowship studying the genetics of auto-immune diseases, and entered private practice in 1988. Since then, she has continued to pursue her interests in the diagnosis and treatment of chronically ill patients. Dr. Fein maintains a private practice in West Caldwell, New Jersey.

Dr. Fein is active in the Lyme disease community. She has lectured at conferences and written journal articles on topics related to Lyme disease. She has served on a New Jersey legislative task force and is medical director for the Pennsylvania Lyme Disease Society and the Greater Hartford (Connecticut) Lyme Disease Support and Action Group. She is a member of the National Lyme Disease Caucus, a group dedicated to the passing of meaningful federal legislation.